Communication
Assessment
and Intervention
with Infants and Toddlers

Communication
Assessment
and Intervention
with Infants and Toddlers

Barbara Weitzner-Lin, PhD

Associate Professor

Buffalo State College

Buffalo, New York

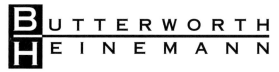

BUTTERWORTH
HEINEMANN

An Imprint of Elsevier

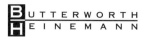

An Imprint of Elsevier

11830 Westline Industrial Drive
St. Louis, Missouri 63146

COMMUNICATION ASSESSMENT AND
INTERVENTION WITH INFANTS AND TODDLERS   ISBN 0-7506-9929-9
Copyright © 2004, Elsevier Inc. All rights reserved.

NOTICE

Speech therapy is an ever-changing field. Standard safety precautions must be followed, but as new research and clinical experience broaden our knowledge, changes in treatment and drug therapy may become necessary or appropriate. Readers are advised to check the most current product information provided by the manufacturer of each drug to be administered to verify the recommended dose, the method and duration of administration, and contraindications. It is the responsibility of the licensed prescriber, relying on experience and knowledge of the patient, to determine dosages and the best treatment for each individual patient. Neither the publisher nor the author assumes any liability for any injury and/or damage to persons or property arising from this publication.

International Standard Book Number 0-7506-9929-9

Publishing Director: Linda Duncan
Managing Editor: Kathy Falk
Associate Developmental Editor: Melissa Kuster Deutsch
Publishing Services Manager: Patricia Tannian
Project Manager: Sharon Corell
Designer: Amy Buxton
All Photos: Courtesy of Kathy Henkel, Bornhava, Buffalo, NY

Printed in United States of America

Last digit is the print number: 9   8   7   6   5   4   3   2   1

This book is dedicated to my family.
B W-L

P R E F A C E

This book provides a framework for assessing the communication abilities of young children (from birth to age 3) and for providing intervention to those children who are communicatively handicapped. This book is intended for early interventionists, specifically for speech-language pathologists. However, the information provided can be adapted for the special educator who provides early intervention services, since communication and language development are the basis for socio-emotional development, the development of inter-personal relationships, and literacy, and are a basic building block for learning. Thus in many instances the text uses the terms early interventionist and speech-language pathologist interchangeably. The book is organized into two main sections. Chapters 1 through 4 provide information about early assess-ment of communicative abilities, and Chapters 5 through 8 provide infor-mation about intervention with children who have communicative handicaps. Each of the two sections ends with a chapter that contains two case studies that translate the theoretical assessment or intervention information into practical clinical applications. The format of the case studies presented in this book serves as a means of translating the presented framework into practical clinical practice. Another feature of these chapters is that when information is given (about assessment or intervention), the rationale for that information is discussed. It is my belief that speech-language pathologists need to be able to justify their practices and procedures to other team members (including families) in a systematic and clear manner.

In the first section, Chapter 1 provides background for the early inter-ventionist about how communication assessment fits into the larger picture of assessing any young child who has special needs. Specifically, this text discusses the importance of including families in the assessment process. I have tried to incorporate information about families in a way that is inclusive of all families; thus this book incorporates information regarding the impact of cultural and ethnic diversity on the family's orientation to early inter-vention. The second chapter discusses the framework of incorporating parents-caregivers as participants in the assessment process and discusses naturalistic methods of obtaining assessment information. A detailed discussion of the components of a comprehensive communication assessment is presented in Chapter 3. Chapter 3 takes as its underlying motivation the belief that a child needs to have a reason to communicate (an intent), something to communi-cate (some content), and lastly but equally important a way in which to communicate the message. This chapter includes a discussion of alternative means of communication as another way in which an infant or toddler can express his or her intent. The use of signs, object boards, or picture boards needs to be incorporated into the assessment process for children who are unable to use speech. Chapter 4 presents the reader with case history infor-mation concerning two infants-toddlers. This chapter is meant to translate the framework discussed in Chapters 1 through 3 to practical clinical practice. First the case history information is given; this is followed by an assessment plan, including justification. The assessment plan describes the additional information that is needed to obtain a complete picture of the child, including methods of obtaining that information. Each case ends with a written report. The format of this chapter is based on the belief that a speech-language pathologist needs to readily present the rationale for all aspects of his or her assessment, as well as to be able to clearly describe this information to caregivers. Although the rationales are written for the professional, they can be easily reformatted for caregivers.

In the second section, Chapter 5 presents a framework for communication intervention with infants and toddlers. It focuses on the use of naturally occurring events in intervention, as well as "best practice" in early intervention. This chapter presents information about different ways in which to involve the family-caregiver in intervention. Chapter 6 presents information about speech-language pathologists working directly with the infant or toddler. The interventionist needs to know when to involve the family and when to implement direct intervention services. Chapter 7 continues the theory presented earlier in the text—that parent or caregiver participation is critical to the development of a young child's communication and language. Chapter 8 illustrates the intervention process, expanding on the case studies presented earlier. Once again this chapter is presented in such a way as to provide the rationale for intervention goals and objectives, as well as family-identified naturally occurring contexts for intervention.

Barbara Weitzner-Lin

ACKNOWLEDGMENTS

Many people have helped and encouraged me in the writing of this book. First of all I would like to thank my students, too numerous to name. Through class discussion they have helped me crystallize my approach to providing early intervention with infants and young children who are communicatively impaired. They will also see an elaboration of case studies they have used to study early communication intervention.

I need to express my thanks to my colleagues who have encouraged me throughout this process. I would especially like to thank Dr. Dolores Battle for starting me on this journey and for her continuous encouragement.

I need to thank the professionals at Bornhava for taking such wonderful pictures of the children. Thank you—Barbara Jo for allowing the pictures to be taken, Kathy for taking such fantastic pictures, and Tammy, for being a friend and colleague whose efforts have gone beyond my expectations. A special thank you goes to the parents, who allowed their children to be a special part of this book.

I need to thank the professionals at Butterworth Heinemann and Elsevier who have been supportive through the year, especially Melissa Kuster, Sharon Corell, and Kathy Falk (and anyone else behind the scenes) for their help in seeing this project come to fruition.

Finally, I need to express my appreciation to my husband, Bill, and children, Jacob and Rebekah, for their love and support. I would particularly like to thank my husband for his constant support of this project, his love, and most important, for being my primary reader and editor.

C O N T E N T S

Overview of Infant-Toddler Assessment and Intervention

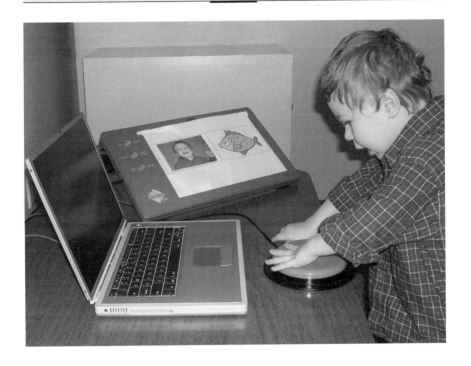

OUTLINE

Sue P. gave birth to her first child, Joshua, but her joy was short-lived when she saw the concerned look on her doctor's face. The words "I'm sorry, but your baby has Down syndrome" still sting. The later news that her son had a heart defect along with other physical abnormalities made the news even more difficult to accept. Sue and her husband, Mike, knew little about the genetic abnormality that had suddenly become a reality in their lives. It was also difficult when family and friends found out about Joshua's birth and did not congratulate the family on the arrival of their first child. Friends and family alike had a difficult time making positive comments about the lovable and charming baby that was now part of Mike and Sue's lives. Sue and Mike are trying to adjust, but they have many questions and worries about the future. These parents want to see their adorable son live a useful life.

Brandon, who is a bright, curious, brown-eyed youngster, is always into everything. When his babbling did not progress beyond engaging in inter-active vocalizations at the age of 24 months, his parents became concerned. Test results obtained by the pediatrician and an audiologist indicated that Brandon had a moderate hearing deficit in both ears and that his hearing problem was further complicated by otitis media (fluid in the middle ear). Brandon, who hears only very loud noises, will need medical intervention for the otitis media and special help to develop communication skills. This family has questions about the medical ramifications of Brandon's hearing problems as well as how Brandon will communicate and the impact his hearing problems and communication delay will have on his learning.

Rena was born at 26 weeks gestation, weighing 880 g. She remained in a neonatal intensive care unit for most of the 10 weeks of her hospital stay. She had an intercerebral hemorrhage and severe hyaline membrane disease. She also had episodes of apnea bradycardia and was sent home with an apnea monitor. Rena's mother has concerns and questions about her development.

Joshua, Brandon, Rena, and other infants and toddlers with conditions similar to theirs are the focus of this book. Because families are systems in which each member has an impact on the others and on the system as a whole, the births and lives of these children have had an impact on their families, just as their families have had an impact on the infants and toddlers. Each of these children's disabilities has affected the family system, as well as the interactions of each child. These children all have a communication problem or a potential communication problem that will affect their ability to bond and interact with their caregivers, to develop social relations with others, to express their wants and needs, to interact with and learn from their environment, and, ultimately, to function independently as they age. Because of this, these three children and their families would benefit from early intervention (EI) services and in particular from communication intervention.

This chapter provides background for the early interventionist and explains how communication assessment and intervention are integral parts of the EI system. It also provides background on important concepts in EI that cross professional disciplines, such as involvement of families and caregivers in the intervention process, team makeup, and service delivery. In this chapter the populations of infants and toddlers with special needs who would benefit from EI services will be reviewed. In addition, information about which children might be candidates for an early communication assessment is presented. A discussion is also included of the impact of cultural diversity on the family's orientation to early assessment and intervention.

RATIONALE AND LEGAL ISSUES IN EARLY INTERVENTION

The Education of the Handicapped Act Amendments P.L. 99-457 of 1986 mandated that states establish comprehensive services for infants and toddlers with disabilities and for their families. The programs established in P.L. 99-457 have been included in the reauthorization of the Individual with Disabilities Education Act. This legislation dramatically changed what services were available to handicapped infants and toddlers and their families, as well as how these services were provided. The law specified that qualified professionals complete the assessment and evaluation, and that a multidisciplinary team perform these services. The legislation referred to evaluation as "the procedures used to determine a child's initial and continuing eligibility for services" (Fewell, 1991, p. 166). Assessment referred to "ongoing procedures used throughout the period of a child's eligibility to identify: (a) the child's unique needs, (b) the family's strengths and needs related to development of the child, and (c) the nature and the extent of the early intervention services needed by the child and the child's family" (Fewell, 1991, p. 166) to meet the needs identified in the evaluation process. Therefore, assessment is completed to do the following:

- Identify children who are likely to be members of groups at risk for health or developmental problems (screening).
- Confirm the presence and extent of a disability (diagnosis).
- Determine appropriate remediation (program planning).
- Ascertain a child's relative knowledge of specific skills and information (readiness tests).
- Demonstrate the extent of a child's previous accomplishments (achievement tests) (Greenspan & Meisels, 1996, p. 12).

Evaluation and assessment of the child must describe the child's functioning in the developmental areas of (1) cognitive development, (2) physical development, (3) language and speech development, (4) psychosocial development, and (5) self-help skills. Part C of the Amendments to the Individuals with Disabilities Education Act (IDEA: P.L. 105-17; 1997) further strengthens the requirements that services be provided to the child in the context of the family.

P.L. 99-457 did more than mandate services for handicapped children from birth to 3 years of age and their families; it also had a philosophical impact on how these services are provided. The legislation emphasized "the interconnections between the children, their families, and the community, and provides guidelines for interdisciplinary collaboration" (Crais, 1992, p. 34). Family members are viewed as primary decision makers in the legislation. The professionals and family collaborate to determine the family's desired outcomes of intervention, as well as to determine the family's resources, concerns, and priorities that might have an impact on the services provided.

FAMILY-CENTERED PRACTICE

Family-centered practice is a philosophical orientation that has been stated to be the foundation of "best practices" in EI (Baird & Petersen, 1997; Crais, 1992; Mahoney & Wheeden, 1997). McWilliam (1996a) identifies six underlying principles of family-centered practice. These include: (1) viewing the family as the unit of service delivery, (2) recognizing child's and family's strengths, (3) responding to family-identified priorities, (4) individualizing service delivery, (5) responding to the changing priorities of families, and (6) supporting family values and lifestyles (p. 2).

SERVICE DELIVERY

The literature typically describes three models of team functioning as a mechanism of providing services to infants and toddlers and their families. The typical models described include the multidisciplinary, interdisciplinary, and transdisciplinary models. Further examination of the literature indicates that there are more possible ways by which teams can function. Donahue-Kilburg (1992) reports four possible means to provide services, with the fourth being the provision of independent services—when professionals work independently without collaboration. More recently, Briggs (1997) elaborated on a systems theory approach for team functioning. In this systems approach, Briggs expands on systems theory and applies this approach to team functioning. She describes the systems approach as it applies to families and expands systems theory in an attempt to mesh the family system and the system of service delivery. The three major service delivery models (multidisciplinary, interdisciplinary, and transdisciplinary) will be further described, with a focus on the family's involvement.

Multidisciplinary
Multidisciplinary teams involve a variety of professional disciplines. These professionals do independent evaluations and decide if the child needs

intervention in the specific discipline. Hence there is little coordination of the recommendations given to the family, and in fact the family may be given conflicting information from the variety of professionals providing service to the child. Bagnato and Neisworth (1991) indicate that this is an "inadequate model" of service delivery. The inadequacies can be examined from the viewpoint of the family, as well as from the perspective of the professionals involved.

From the family's perspective:

- The family may be interacting with many professionals and receiving a lot of information that might be conflicting.
- Parents do not know who to direct their questions to.
- The family may feel as if they have no input, unless they find a professional who values their input.
- The family may feel overwhelmed and threatened by the number of individuals involved with their child as well as by the demands made on the family.
- Scheduling conflicts may exist as each professional representative vies for specific times with the child.
- There may be overlap of services.

From the professional's viewpoint:

- He or she may be unaware of the other disciplines involved.
- There may be a lack of communication among professionals leading to a very narrow view of the child.
- It may be more difficult for the professional to meet established outcomes because there is no sharing of resources and information.

Interdisciplinary

The interdisciplinary team, on the other hand, has established lines of communication among professionals. There is a greater degree of cooperation among the professionals involved, and the family is often considered part of the team. Typically, the different disciplines assess the child independently; then the team comes together to present the family with a more cohesive view of the child for intervention planning purposes. Professionals from specific disciplines may still provide discipline specific intervention; however, there is more cooperative planning (Briggs, 1997; Costarides, Shulman, Trimm, & Brady, 1998; Rossetti, 1990). The professional is providing intervention services from his or her discipline's perspective but does look to the other professionals for support and to share information. This model still has some inadequacies, from both the family's and the professional's perspective.

From the family's perspective:

- There is no team leader. As a result, there is no one to direct questions to concerning overall management concerns.
- Conflicting opinions are still voiced to the family.
- Family members are not considered full team members.
- There still may be too many professionals involved.

From the professional's perspective:

- There is no team leader.
- An intervention program may not be fully integrated.
- A significant amount of time is spent in team meetings.

Transdisciplinary

The family is considered an integral member of the transdisciplinary team. The team crosses disciplinary boundaries so that all members can function as an integrated unit. All members of the transdisciplinary team complete the assessment in a format called an *arena assessment*. An arena assessment has all team members observe the child while interacting with either a family member or a team member. The whole team develops an integrated service plan, and the key to this service plan is that it is developed through consensus or collaboration with the family. Typically, a case manager, coordinator of care, or primary service provider implements the service plan with the family. Team members share the responsibility for the success of the service plan by providing formal and informal support to the family and the primary service provider (McGonigel, Woodruff, & Roszmann-Millican, 1994). Although many consider the transdisciplinary model the ideal model in the provision of EI services, it, too, may have some inadequacies for the family and the professional.

From the family's perspective:

- The professional may be providing service beyond his or her expertise.
- There is no buffer in case of a personality conflict between the family and the primary service provider.

From the professional's perspective:

- Some professionals may have an inadequate understanding of other professionals' disciplines.
- Extra effort may be needed to learn about other disciplines.
- Personality clashes may occur.
- May not feel comfortable giving up one's professional role
- Time must be set aside for team members to build trusting and effective working relationships.

INDIVIDUALIZED FAMILY SERVICE PLANS

P.L. 99-457 instituted a requirement that, for each child being serviced, a written document, the Individualized Family Service Plan (IFSP), must be developed. The IFSP can be considered the map of the services to be provided to the child and his or her family. This map must indicate the services that are needed to maximize the child's development and enable the family to influence their child's development. Fewell, Snyder, Sexton, Bertrand, and Hockless (1991) indicated that the following information must be included in the IFSP:

- Information about the child's current status.
- Information about the family (resources, priorities, and concerns).
- Specific intervention services needed to meet the child's needs.
- Expected outcomes.
- Duration of service and dates of initiation.
- Designated case manager.
- Transition services.

The law does not specify a format for the IFSP but allows the assessment teams to develop what works best for them (McGonigel, Kaufman, & Johnson,

1991). In a family-centered practice these elements should result in a plan that will work effectively. McWilliam (1996b) indicates that the best IFSPs are those that are used by families and professionals. McWilliam further described the characteristics of IFSPs that are considered useful. These characteristics include the following:

- Parents understand and agree with the content.
- Parents have a sense of ownership of the plan that is developed.
- The plan includes goals that are important to the family.
- Activities for accomplishing goals are enjoyable for the child and the family.
- Activities are embedded in daily routines.
- There is a high likelihood of accomplishing goals within a relatively short time.
- Resources are available and accessible for implementing activities (e.g., time, money, emotional support, energy, space, materials).
- The intervention plan is amenable to frequent revisions and updating.
- The plan is reviewed frequently and planning is a continuous process.
- The written plan passes the "piggy magnet test" (is short, concise, and can be mounted on the refrigerator with a magnet) (p.113).

McWilliam, Ferguson, Harbin, Porter, Munn & Vandiviere (1998) further indicate that IFSPs should reflect what the family wants in that they should include strategies that match outcomes, specify the family's role, and be inclusive. McWilliam et al. (1998) also indicate that the IFSP should be clearly written (positively, specifically, and nonjudgmentally). Lastly, these authors indicate that the IFSP should be functional (i.e., be necessary for success, be appropriate to context or incorporated into everyday routines and events, and be written in the active voice).

INFANTS AND TODDLERS: WHO MIGHT BENEFIT?

Tjossem (1976) described three categories of infants vulnerable to developmental delay or disorder and in need of EI services. These categories are: "(1) infants manifesting early appearing aberrant development related to diagnosed medical disorders with established risk for delayed development, (2) infants at environmental risk consequent to depriving life experiences, and (3) infants at biological risk as determined by increased probability for delayed or aberrant development consequent to biological insult" (p. 4). Infants and toddlers with developmental delays are also at risk for a communication delay. In addition to those children at risk for developmental delay concurrent to a communication delay, some children exhibit only a communication delay. Both sets of children are included in the categories described by Tjossem. Since both children with developmental delays in conjunction with communication delays and children with communication delays alone are seen by the early interventionists, understanding the established risk, environmental risk, and biological risk categories is important.

It should be noted that in addition to the categories described below, a series of biological conditions might be specifically related to early language delay. These include heredity, gender, oromotor problems, and a history of early otitis media. Heredity could be considered a significant risk factor. In fact, Olswang, Rodriguez, and Timler (1998) indicate that "if one of the toddler's parents or siblings demonstrates persistent language and learning difficulties, the risk of continued language delay is increased" (p. 27). Whitehurst, Fischel, Arnold, and Lonigan (1992) indicate that language impairment tends to occur more in males than females, as do other medical problems. Whitehurst et al. (1992) also point out that although not all children with early language delay have oromotor problems, a connection exists between these two conditions in some children with early language impairments. Olswang et al. (1998) indicate that "prolonged, untreated, otitis media places a child at greater risk of continued language delay" (p.28). Therefore these factors should alert the early interventionist that early communicative intervention might be warranted.

Established Risk Factors

Infants and toddlers at established risk are those who have a variety of medical conditions that are known to present developmental delay (with a concurrent communication delay or a communication delay alone). Refer to Table 1-1 for established risk conditions. Included in the established risk category are genetic and metabolic conditions. Chromosomal anomalies and genetic disorders that are associated with established risk for developmental delay include conditions such as trisomy 21, cri du chat syndrome, and fragile X syndrome. Inborn errors in metabolism (metabolic disorders) also may have established risk for developmental functioning. Phenylketonuria, thyroid disorders (such as hypothyroidism), and mucopolysaccharidoses (such as Hunter syndrome) are included in metabolic disorders.

Also included in the category of established risk would be a variety of neurological disorders that typically present developmental delay. These conditions or disorders may have been the result of a prenatal, perinatal, or postnatal impact on the central nervous system (CNS) that has resulted in a neurological disorder. The metabolic disorders and genetic disorders described above are included in the prenatal causes of CNS dysfunction. Perinatal conditions such as asphyxia have resulted in cerebral palsy (a dysfunction of central nervous system). Postnatal etiologic factors include CNS infections (meningitis), accidents (head trauma from vehicular accidents or child abuse), and lead toxicity, all of which carry established risk for developmental disorders (Rubin, 1990). Infants and toddlers who have congenital malformations, sensory disorders, or both are also at established risk. Congenital malformations include such conditions as cleft palate, Treacher Collins syndrome, and spina bifida. Developmental disorders or associated communication disorders are often concurrent with many of these conditions. Sensory disorders include visual and auditory impairments.

Environmental and Biological Risk Factors

Environmental risk and biological risk conditions have been described as including infants and toddlers who are at risk for a developmental delay (which may include a communication delay). Refer to Table 1-2 for a listing of biological and environmental risk factors. Infants and toddlers who may be at biological risk are those whose central and peripheral nervous systems

Table 1-1	*Established risk conditions*
ESTABLISHED RISK POTENTIAL	MANIFESTATIONS
Chromosomal Anomalies or Genetic Disorders	Cri-du chat
	Trisomy 18
	Cockayne syndrome
	Waardenbburg syndrome
	Trisomy 21 (Down Syndrome)
	Fragile X syndrome
	Laurence-Moon-Bardet-Biedl syndrome
	Cerebro-hepato-renal syndrome
Neurological Disorders	Cerebral Palsy
	Progressive muscular dystrophy
	Paralysis
	Intercranial hemorrhage
	Werdnig Hoffman disease
	Neurofibromatosis
	Intercranial tumors
	Seizure disorder
	Kernicterus
	Myasthenia Congenita
	Wilson disease
	Kuelberg-Welander disease
	Schildre disease
	Sturge-Weber syndrome
	Head and spinal cord injury
Congenital Malformations	Patent ductus arterilsis
	Transposition of great arteries
	Noonan syndrome
	Potter syndrome
	Spina Bifida
	Cleft palate
	Hyoplastic mandible
	Treacher Collins syndrome
	Microcephaly
Inborn Errors in Metabolism	Hunter syndrome
	Marqulo syndrome
	Maple syrup urine disease
	Galactosemia
	Neimann-Pick disease
	Hurler-Schele syndrome
	Tay-Sachs disease
	Infant PKU
	Glycogen storage disease
	Hyperpituitary-Hypopituitary disease
Sensory Disorders	Visual impairment-blindness
	Hearing loss
	Retinopathy of prematurity
	Congenital cataract

| Table 1-2 | *Biological and environmental risk factors* |

RISK FACTOR	CAUSES
Biological Risk	
Severe Toxic Exposure	Cocaine and other drugs
	Maternal PKU
	Fetal alcohol syndrome
	Lead-mercury poisoning
Severe Infectious Disease	Cytomegalovirus (CMV)
	HIV+
	Syphilis
	Bacterial meningitis
	Poliomyelitis
	Herpes
	Rubella
	Toxoplasmosis
	Encephalitis
	Viral meningitis
Birth Process	Premature birth with increased risk of respiratory disorders
	Intraventricular hemorrhage
Environmental Risk	
Maternal-Caregiver Factors	Caregiver with chronic or severe illness
	Caregiver with mental illness
	Caregiver with developmental disability, mental retardation
	Adolescent mother, limited prenatal care, etc.
Psychosocial factors	Caregiver–child separation
	Lack of stable residence
	Physical or social isolation
	Family in crisis

experienced an incident from the time of conception forward that affected development. Several prenatal events are known to result in a high risk for developmental problems; these include substance abuse during pregnancy and a variety of maternal infections during pregnancy. Substance abuse includes the extensive use of alcohol, tobacco, and a variety of prescribed or illicit medications taken during pregnancy.

The extensive use of alcohol during pregnancy produces fetal alcohol syndrome (FAS), which is the leading cause of mental retardation in the United States (Costarides, Shulman, Trimm & Brady, 1998). Exposure to alcohol that does not result in FAS still can cause behavioral, attention, and learning problems. Use of tobacco during pregnancy can cause intrauterine growth retardation, which can result in lower than expected birth weight. Lower than expected birth weight increases risk for developmental problems in all domains. Likewise, exposure to a variety of illegal substances (cocaine) and prescribed medications can result in developmental problems.

The birth process itself can leave an infant at biological risk for developmental disorders. Prematurity is one of the most significant factors in infant morbidity and mortality (Costarides et al., 1998). Premature birth increases the infant's risk for respiratory disorders (respiratory distress syndrome), intraventricular hemorrhage, and exposure to ototoxic drugs, all of which can increase the infant's chances of a developmental delay.

Maternal infections have also been associated with developmental delay or disorders. Maternal infections include cytomegalovirus, human immuno-deficiency virus, and rubella.

Environmental risk factors that result in the deprivation of life experiences also must be taken into consideration. This group of risk factors includes maternal or caregiver factors and psychosocial factors.

The presence of one or more of the environmental and biological risk factors may not in itself result in a developmental disorder; it is the layering of these risk factors that has been associated with increased likelihood of a developmental delay. Rossetti (2001) indicates that there is a continuum of risk factors that make prognosis statements difficult to formulate. The early interventionist needs to be aware of the developmental expectations of various populations of infants and toddlers who are at risk for developmental delay and the "links between risk factors presented and how they interact and contribute to communication delay, general developmental performance, and later school achievement" (p. 38).

RESPECTING CULTURAL DIVERSITY

The United States has been described as a melting pot, but rather than representing a blending together of differences, the United States is presently celebrating those differences and realizing that there are many fabrics of American life. The effectiveness of family-centered EI requires that the EI professional be able to meet the needs of culturally and linguistically diverse families as well as meeting the special needs of the child. To do so requires that the professional interact with the family in a manner that is sensitive to the culture and language background of the family. Chan (1990) indicates that professionals in EI need to be culturally competent in order to be effective in providing family-centered services to families from culturally and linguistically diverse backgrounds. Cultural competence refers to the way in which the early interventionist thinks and behaves that enables that professional to work effectively with members of diverse cultural, linguistic, and ethnic groups. Chan indicates that cultural competence includes the following:

- Self-awareness and awareness of the "dynamics of difference" (including understanding "culture" and its function in human behavior).
- Knowledge of culture-specific information pertaining to various ethnic groups.
- Skills needed to engage in successful cross-cultural interactions with culturally diverse populations (p. 8).

Self-awareness is the understanding of one's own culture (Chan, 1990; Lynch, 1998), including behaviors, customs, and habits that are culturally based. After gaining an understanding of one's own culture, an individual can begin to recognize and appreciate the diversity of families from different cultures. Lynch (1998) indicates that individuals who are part of mainstream culture are probably the least aware of the ways in which culture affects their behavior and interactions.

Once awareness is achieved, the professional should obtain knowledge of culture-specific information (Chan, 1990). Lynch (1998) indicates that the most effective ways of obtaining this information are: (1) learning through books, the arts, and technology; (2) talking and working with individuals from the culture who can act as cultural guides or mediators; (3) participating in the daily life of another culture; and (4) learning the language of the other culture (p. 55).

Hanson, Lynch, and Wayman (1990) further indicate that the EI professional should obtain information about the specific cultures in the community through ethnographic study of the community. These authors indicate that the professional needs to (1) describe the ethnic group with which the family identifies, (2) identify the social organizations of the ethnic community, (3) describe the prevailing belief system within the ethnic community, (4) learn about the history of the ethnic group and current events that directly and indirectly affect the family, (5) determine how members of the community gain access and use social services, and (6) identify the attitudes of the ethnic community with regard to seeking help.

A caution for early interventionists when learning about different cultures is to not stereotype. The EI professional "should not stereotype or prejudge a family on the basis of the family's ethnicity and culture. Each individual and each family will have had contact with external cultures. Such contact increases the cultural and linguistic diversity among families" (Anderson, 1991, pp. 9-10). The contact does more than to increase the diversity; it also impacts the degree to which the family will identify with and practice traditional customs and beliefs.

To develop the skills needed to engage in successful cross-cultural interactions, interventionists must have specific information related to cultural views of children and child rearing practices, family roles and structure, views of disability and its causes, health and healing practices, and views of change and intervention (Hanson et al., 1990). Knowledge of child-rearing practices is crucial for the EI professional because the intervention strategies offered by the professional may be in conflict with the practices of a specific family. The roles of family members will affect family-centered services, since the professional needs to know who the family decision maker is and who is closest to the child. The family's view on disability may also affect the services accepted and provided. Many cultures attribute disability to spiritual causes or view it as the family's fate and something that can't be helped. The family's views of causation of disability will also affect how that family traditionally deals with the child with special needs. The family may select to do nothing, attributing the circumstance to "fate," or they may prefer to consult healers, elders, or both. The EI professionals should be familiar with this information because it will affect the types of services the family may be willing to accept, as well as the type of information the family is willing to share with the EI professional.

Professionals working with families from diverse cultures also need to be aware that there are various aspects of communication, such as the amount of information that is transmitted through words versus the amount of information transmitted through nonverbal communication or through read-ing the situation. Awareness of such issues will enhance the communication between the EI professional and the family.

IMPACT OF THE FAMILY'S CULTURE ON THEIR ATTITUDE TOWARD THE HANDICAPPED AND EARLY INTERVENTION

Cultural influences are an integral part of our lives. A family's culture (values and beliefs) will affect that family's views of every aspect of life, including the identification of a child with a disability. Interaction styles, family structure, child rearing practices, treatment practices, and language may also differ from culture to culture. Even within the same culture there may be differences from family to family. The language that a child acquires mirrors the language behaviors, norms, and expectations of the family (Battle, 1997). The family's notion of disability will also have an impact on their attitude about the need for EI and on the role the family takes in the intervention process. Inherent in P.L. 99-457 is the mandatory involvement of families in the intervention process; thus it is especially important to consider the family's views and beliefs when implementing a family-centered program. The early inter-ventionist needs to recognize that some families may be surprised by the extent of parent–professional collaboration that is expected in intervention programs. The EI professional must realize that direct confrontation and questioning or informal and indirect questioning concerning personal matters such as their child's development and birth history, communication, family issues, or other personal information may be improper and inappropriate in the family's culture (Hanson, 1998). The family's perspective on questioning is only one interaction practice that may affect the EI process. How infor-mation is collected (oral or written formats), the person to whom inquiries are directed (mother, father, or elder), as well as views of independence and privacy must all be taken into consideration (Hanson, 1998). There are additional influences on families other than their cultural identification, including socioeconomic status, educational level, occupation, and personal experience.

The speech and language pathologist (as well as other EI professionals) needs to understand (1) that the family's culture has an influence on their expectation of communicative competence and communication practices and (2) that feeding practices will vary, which in turn will affect intervention practices. A complement to the family's expectations of communication competence is the culture's (family's) identification of a communication disorder. Communication and its disorders must be viewed from a cultural perspective. Paul (2001) indicates that there may be a mismatch between the communicative expectations of the mainstream culture and the commu-nication style of specific cultures. The interventionists need to determine if there is a mismatch in expectations or if there is a communication problem. Specific communication practices vary from culture to culture. For example, methods of greeting (formal versus informal), degree of eye contact when interacting, amount of social distance, and use of gestures may vary from culture to culture and should be considered. Likewise, feeding practices are cultural phenomena; thus the cultural attitudes about meal times will influence whether language activities can be incorporated during this event, as well as the family's responsiveness to suggestions to alter feeding practices as part of an intervention program.

Implicit in understanding the family's attitude toward EI is (as previously indicated) that the professional needs to have information about the socio-cultural influences on the family's values and beliefs that might affect EI. If the professional does not have that information, a cultural informant may be needed to supply that information and to serve as a link between the family and the professional. The cultural informant must be competent in interpreting the contexts, values, and meaning of the language and behaviors used by the family, as well as by the EI professional (Barrera, 1996). For example, the cultural informant must be able to recognize and interpret a mother's desire, even insistence, that a specific appointment time for a home visit be established not as presenting an obstacle but as a way to ensure that her husband can be home at the designated time to monitor the unfamiliar visitors to his home.

NONDISCRIMINATORY ASSESSMENT

P.L. 99-457 indicated that assessment of infants and toddlers must be nondiscriminatory. The law specified that all tests and other procedures be administered in the child's or the parent's native language or their preferred mode of communication (*Federal Register*, 1989, reported in Fewell, 1991). Thus part of an EI assessment must include a determination of the family's (and the child's) dominant language (or preferred language). If it is not possible to administer the test in the family's (child's) dominant or preferred language, the use of an interpreter (cultural informant) may facilitate the evaluation/assessment process. Barrera (1996) indicates that the responsibility of a cultural informant is to "assist service providers in becoming aware of any unfamiliar values, behaviors, language, or rules that are part of the family's environment and to assist the family and the child in becoming familiar with any unfamiliar values, beliefs, language or rules that are part of the assessment and intervention environment" (p. 77). The cultural informant or translator must be bilingual, proficient in both the language of the child or family and that of the assessment professionals. The cultural informant or translator also needs to be competent in interpreting the contexts, values, and meaning of the language and behavior used (Barrera, 1996). Lynch (1998) indicates that the early interventionist should be cautious when working with an interpreter. If the interpreter is a family member, that person may censor information in an effort to "protect" the family. If using a nonfamily member the interventionist should respect the family's right to privacy and their choice of interpreter. An interpreter can facilitate communication between the early interventionist and the family when the language of the family is not that of the interventionist, and the interpreter can also translate test materials into the family's or child's dominant language. Cheng (1993) cautioned against the use of an interpreter to translate a standardized test into the child's dominant language. Translation of a test violates the test's standardization; equally (if not more) important is that just because a concept (or word) is translated does not mean that the concept (or word) is important in the individual's language or culture. In addition, test procedures and materials should not be culturally or racially discriminatory.

WHY DO SPEECH–LANGUAGE PATHOLOGISTS GET INVOLVED IN EARLY INTERVENTION?

Speech–language pathologists are professionals who are trained to work with individuals with communication disorders. Communication skills are crucial to many areas of early childhood development, and these skills lay the foundation for the child's ability to develop relationships, to learn from others, to develop the ability to share knowledge and past experiences, as well as to develop literacy. Language skills serve as the basis for academic achievement. Speech–language pathologists are on the EI team to provide services to infants and toddlers who may have a communication or a speech–language delay, so that these children can develop communication skills as a foundation for subsequent school achievement. P.L. 99-457, the amendment to Title 1 of the Education of the Handicapped Act (retitled as IDEA in 1990), in Part H (now retitled Part C of IDEA, Infants and Toddlers with Disabilities Program) of that law, included speech–language pathologists as the professionals to provide speech and language services.

Children such as Joshua have a condition that puts them at risk for a communication delay. The research supports the view that these children do in fact have difficulty learning to communicate. The EI team working with Joshua needs to pay special attention to his communication. Infants such as Brandon have a speech and language impairment secondary to a history of hearing loss. However, the research is unclear on whether recurrent otitis media is enough of a risk factor to cause a significant speech and language delay. Children such as Brandon may be among the five children out of every 100 who will have significant language delays and disabilities (*Communication Facts*, 2002). Brandon and others like him need to be provided with early speech and language services to ensure that they develop a communication system as an entrance into society and learning. Infants such as Rena are also at risk for a communication delay. The cerebral hemorrhage may impact motor functioning, which in turn impacts oral motor development and the ability to develop speech. Rena and others like her need speech and language services to develop their communication system.

REFERENCES

Anderson, N. B. (1991). Understanding cultural diversity. *American Journal of Speech Language Pathology*, September, 9-10.

Bagnato, S. J., & Neisworth, J. T. (1991). *Assessment for early intervention: Best practices for professionals*. New York: Guilford Press.

Baird, S., & Peterson, J. (1997). Seeking a comfortable fit between family-centered philosophy and infant–parent interaction in early intervention: Time for a paradigm shift? *Topics in Early Childhood Special Education, 17*(2), 139-164.

Barrera, I. (1996). Thoughts on the assessment of young children whose sociocultural background is unfamiliar to the assessor. In S. Meisels & E. Fenichel (Eds.), *New visions for the assessment of infants and young children* (pp. 69-84). Washington, D.C.: Zero to Three.

Battle, D. E. (1997). Language and communication disorders in culturally and linguistically diverse children. In D. K. Bernstein & E. Tiegerman-Farber (Eds.), *Language and communication disorders in children* (4th Ed.) (pp. 382-409). Boston: Allyn & Bacon.

Briggs, M. H. (1997). A systems model for early intervention teams. *Infants and Young Children, 9*(3), 69-77.

Chan, S. (1990). Early intervention with culturally diverse families of infants and toddlers with disabilities. *Infants and Young Children, 3*(2), 78-87.

Cheng, L. (1993). Asian–American cultures. In D. E. Battle (Ed.), *Communication disorders in multicultural populations* (pp. 38-77). Boston: Andover Medical Publishers.

Communication Facts: Incidence and prevalence of communication disorders and hearing loss in children, 2002 Edition. Retrieved October 13, 2003, from www.asha.org/members/research/reports/children.

Costarides, A. H., Shulman, B. B., Trimm, R. F., & Brady, N. R. (1998). Monitoring at-risk infant and toddler development: A transdisciplinary approach. *Topics in Language Disorders, 18*(3), 1-14.

Crais, E. R. (1992). Best practices with preschoolers: Assessing within the context of a family-centered approach. In J. Damico & W. Secord (Eds.), *Best practices in school speech–language pathology, 2* (pp. 33-42). NY: Psychological Corp.

Donahue-Kilburg, G. (1992). *Family-centered early intervention for communication disorders: Prevention and treatment.* Gaithersburg, MD: Aspen Publications, Inc.

Fewell, R. R. (1991). Trends in the assessment of infants and toddlers with disabilities. *Exceptional Children* (October-November), 166-173.

Fewell, R. R., Snyder, P., Sexton, D., & Hockless, M. F. (1991). Implementing IFSPs in Louisiana: Different formats for family-centered practices under Part H. *Topics in Early Childhood Special Education, 11*(3), 54-65.

Greenspan, S. I., & Meisels, S. J. (1996). Toward a new vision for the developmental assessment of infants and young children. In S. J. Meisels & E. Fenichel (Eds.), *New visions for the developmental assessment of infants and young children* (pp. 11-26). Washington, D.C.: Zero to Three.

Hanson, M. J. (1998). Ethnic, cultural, and language diversity in intervention settings. In E. W. Lynch & M. J. Hanson (Eds.), *Developing cross-cultural competence: A guide for working with children and their families* (2nd Ed.) (pp. 3-22). Baltimore: Paul H. Brookes Publishing Co.

Hanson, M. J., Lynch, E. W., & Wayman, K. I. (1990). Honoring the cultural diversity of families when gathering data. *Topics in Early Childhood Special Education, 10*(1), 112-131.

Lynch, E. W. (1998). Developing cross-cultural competence. In E. W. Lynch & M. J. Hanson (Eds.), *Developing cross-cultural competence: A guide for working with children and their families* (2nd Ed.) (pp. 47-89). Baltimore: Paul H. Brookes Publishing Co.

Lynch, E. W., & Hanson, M. J. (1998). *Developing cross-cultural competence: A guide for working with children and their families* (2nd Ed). Baltimore: Paul H. Brookes Publishing Co.

Mahoney, G., & Wheeden, C. A. (1997). Parent–child interaction: The foundation for family-centered early intervention practice—A response to Baird and Peterson. *Topics in Early Childhood Special Education, 17*(2), 165-187.

McGonigel, M. J., Kaufman, R. K., & Johnson, B. H. (1991). *Guidelines and recommended practices for the individualized family service plan* (2nd Ed.). Bethesda: Association for the Care of Children's Health.

McGonigel, M. J., Woodruff, G., & Roszmann-Millican, M. (1994). The transdisciplinary team: A model for family-centered early intervention. In L. J. Johnson, R. J. Gallagher, M. J. LaMontagne, J. B. Jordan, J. J. Gallagher, P. L. Hutinger, & M. B. Karnes (Eds.), *Meeting early intervention challenges: Issues from birth to three* (2nd Ed.) (pp. 95-131). Baltimore: Paul H. Brookes Publishing Co.

McWilliam, P. J. (1996a). Family-centered practices in early intervention. In P. J. McWilliam, P. J. Winton & E. R. Crais (Eds.) *Practical strategies for family-centered intervention* (pp. 1-14). San Diego, CA: Singular Publishing Group.

McWilliam, P. J. (1996b). Family-centered intervention planning. In P. J. McWilliam, P. J. Winton & E. R. Crais (Eds.) *Practical strategies for family-centered intervention* (pp. 97-123). San Diego, CA: Singular Publishing Group.

McWilliam, R. A., Ferguson, A., Harbin, G. L., Porter, P., Munn, D., & Vandiviere, P. (1998). The family-centeredness of Individualized Family Service Plans. *Topics in Early Childhood Special Education, 18*(2), 69-82.

Olswang, L. B., Rodriguez, B., & Timler, G. (1998). Recommending intervention for toddlers with specific language learning difficulties: We may not have all the answers, but we know a lot. *American Journal of Speech–Language Pathology, 3*(7), 23-32.

Paul, R. (2001). *Language disorders from infancy through adolescence: Assessment and intervention* (2nd Ed). St. Louis, MO: Mosby.

Rossetti, L. (1990). *Infant–toddler assessment: An interdisciplinary approach.* Boston: College-Hill Press.

Rossetti, L. (2001). Populations at risk for communication delay. In L. Rossetti (Ed.), *Communication intervention: Birth to three* (pp. 1-43). San Diego: Singular Publishing Group.

Rubin, I. L. (1990). Etiology of developmental disabilities. *Infants and young children, 3*(1), 25-32. Also in Blackman, J. A. (Ed.) (1995). *Medical aspects of early intervention.* Gaithersburg, MD: Aspen Publication.

Tjossem, T. (1976). Early intervention: Issues and approaches. In T. Tjossem (Ed.), *Intervention strategies for high risk infants and young children* (pp. 3-33). Baltimore: University Park Press.

Whitehurst, G. J., Fischel, J. E., Arnold, D. S., & Lonigan, C. L. (1992). Evaluating outcomes with children with expressive language delay. In S. Warren & J. Reichle (Eds.), *Causes and effects in communication and language intervention* (pp. 277-313). Baltimore: Paul H. Brookes Publishing Co.

CHAPTER 2

Framework for Assessing Communication of Infants and Toddlers

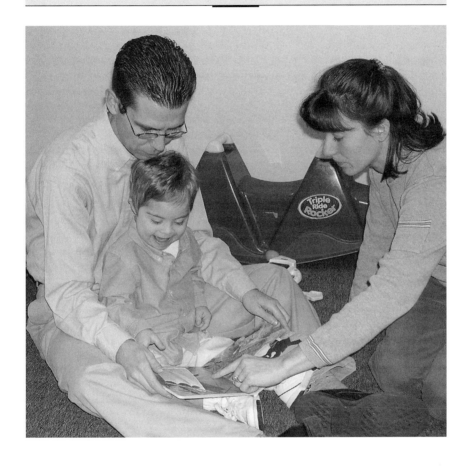

OUTLINE

This chapter discusses a framework for incorporating parents and caregivers as participants in the assessment process and discusses naturalistic methods of obtaining assessment information. The newer framework of incorporating parents and caregivers in the assessment process is contrasted with a more traditional model of assessment, which is professionally driven. The newer approach is family centered, in which the family, not the professional, is the decision maker. Briggs (1998) recognizes that an infant's or toddler's communicative change should occur in the context of the family and that to achieve such an end, the roles of both the professional and family members involved also must change. The professional's role shifts from that of agent of change to facilitator, and the family's role is expanded, with the family moving from receiver of information to catalyst of change.

Within this newer family-driven framework there are a variety of goals that must be met for the assessment to be effective. The goals of the assessment must be clearly delineated and accepted by those involved in the process. When assessing young children the goals of the assessment must be ones that are, at a minimum, acceptable to the family of the child being assessed, as well as to the professionals who are involved. For an assessment of the speech and language or communication abilities of the young child to be effective, the assumptions listed in Box 2-1 must be taken into consideration. In addition to these assumptions, the speech–language professional must always remember that there is variation in the normal sequence of communication development in typical young children.

Box 2-1	*Assumptions underlying early intervention*

1. Family centered
2. Ecologically based
3. Individualized and incorporating multiple measures
4. Culturally sensitive and nondiscriminatory
5. Enabling and empowering
6. Based on family concerns
7. Coordinated with other community agencies
8. Normalized
9. Involves professionals from other disciplines
10. Comprehensive

Compiled from Richard, N. B., & Schiefelbusch, R. L. (1990). Assessment. In L. McCormick and R. L. Schiefelbusch (Eds.), *Early language intervention: An introduction* (2nd Ed.). Columbus, OH: Merrill Publishing Co.; Crais, E. R. (1994). *Increasing family participation in the assessment of children birth to five*. Chicago: Riverside Publishing Co.; Weitzner-Lin, B. (1992). Infants and toddlers: Contemporary assessment issues. Weitzner-Lin, B. & Crais, E. (Eds.), *Infants and toddlers*. Miniseminar. New York State Speech Language and Hearing Association, Kiamesha Lake, NY, April 1992.

ASSUMPTIONS UNDERLYING EARLY INTERVENTION

Family Centered

The first assumption underlying effective early intervention is that effective assessment is family centered. Implicit in this assumption is that the roles that professionals, agencies, and families assume during the assessment process will change (Leviton, Mueller, & Kauffman, 1992). Family-centered intervention involves caregivers both as informants and as significant partners in the assessment process. In the past, the role of the caregiver in an assessment was limited to that of provider of information with the information being initiated and gathered by the professionals. Traditionally, caregivers also were receivers of information upon the completion of the assessment. By involving caregivers in the assessment process from the beginning, professionals can develop a partnership with the family and work toward the family's desired outcomes. Inherent in this is a relationship that involves trust and mutual respect. Miller and Hanft (1998) indicate that a positive alliance between families and professionals should be established to assist in the development of collaborative relationships with families. A more family-centered approach offers families choices in terms of their level of participation (Miller & Hanft, 1998).

Caregivers can have many important roles in the assessment process, ranging from the traditional roles of informant and receiver of information to observer of child behavior, active participant, or examiner or evaluator (Crais, 1994). Other roles family members may assume during the assessment process include narrator, coach, reflector, and elicitor (Miller & Hanft, 1998). Caregivers have been asked to complete various types of assessment and screening protocols, and "concurrent agreement between parent report and professional assessment has been reported to range from 75% to 95%" (Diamond & Squires, 1993, p. 113). Yet despite such reliable findings, parents generally have not been considered to be viable sources of information concerning their children's development and have been excluded from involvement in assessment (Henderson & Meisels, 1994). Caregivers have multiple opportunities to view their children in a variety of situations and contexts and over extended periods of time. Caregivers can thus reliably complete assessment forms such as the *MacArthur Communicative Development Inventories* (Fenson, Dale, Reznick, Thal, Bates, Hartung, Patrick & Reilly, 1993), as well as report on their observations of the child's use of language in the home and in other settings that the assessor cannot observe. Caregivers can also relay information about the child's communication strategies and language abilities when interacting with other significant communicative partners who may not be present during the assessment (spouse, siblings, grandparents, and others). Another reason for our needing to include parents in the assessment process is that young children with handicaps generally do not respond optimally to assessments conducted by strangers (Miller & Hanft, 1998). Thus we need to use family members in order to obtain valid information about children. Another important role that a parent can have in the assessment process is as interpreter of the child's behavior (Henderson & Meisels, 1994). This notion of family involvement in assessment should also be carried into intervention as research on the longitudinal outcomes of parents implementing intervention has found "significant differences in child functioning variables in favor of the child in the home parent training groups" (Eiserman, Weber, & McCoun, 1995, p. 21).

Not only do parents need to be offered a variety of roles in the early intervention process, professionals also need to assume a variety of roles in order to have effective intervention. Professionals must be prepared to assume the following roles: (1) assisting parents in making choices about their roles in intervention; (2) providing direct intervention (or assessment) with children; and (3) helping parents develop skills to provide direct interventions with their children (Eiserman et al., 1995, p. 42).

Ecologically Based

Effective assessment is also ecologically based. This provides us with another reason why it is important to partner with caregivers during the assessment process. To ensure the home ecology, caregivers must be involved in the assessment. Caregivers will also serve as the representative of the larger ecology (that of the neighborhood, community, and culture). The traditional model of assessment by strangers requiring the young child to perform irrelevant tasks in an isolated setting does not provide anyone with a true picture of the child's communication abilities.

Individualized and Incorporating Multiple Measures

Effective assessment is individualized and incorporates multiple measures and multiple sources of information. It is not possible to obtain a well-developed picture of a young child's communication abilities based on one view of the child. In addition, a single standardized evaluation usually does not answer the family's questions (Miller & Hanft, 1998). Information should be provided by the family, by direct observation of the child using his or her communication abilities in natural contexts, and by results of standardized or more formal assessment procedures.

Culturally Sensitive and Nondiscriminatory

Effective assessment is culturally sensitive and nondiscriminatory. Among the principles underlying P.L. 99-457 are the following: "early intervention systems and strategies must reflect a respect for racial, ethnic, and cultural diversity of families and early intervention services should be flexible, accessible, and responsive to family needs" (Chan, 1990, p. 78). The assessment should not penalize the child because of his or her race, gender, or cultural background. Nondiscriminatory assessment, as discussed in P.L. 99-457, indicates that (1) assessment procedures to be administered to the child or the parents should be in their native language (or the family's chosen language), (2) the materials used in assessment should not be discriminatory, and (3) multiple methods must be employed in assessment (Fewell, 1991). For the assessment to be valid, the early interventionist should take into consideration the assessment procedures, materials, instruments, and interactions that reflect the views, values, and expectations of both the interventionist and the family. Only when the values and expectations of both the family and the interventionist are incorporated into the assessment process can the interventionist assume that the information obtained is accurate and valid (Barrera, 1996). Biased assessment may result in a child being labeled as having a disability when in fact the assessment itself contributed to the child's poor performance (Battle, 1997). In a culturally sensitive, family-centered approach, an ethnographic interview allows the evaluators to determine the cultural and environmental influences on the child's development of communication in the home as well as the dimensions of communicative competence important to the family and the culture (Battle, 1997).

Enabling and Empowering

For an assessment to be effective, it must also be enabling and empowering to the family. The process should not place barriers between the family and professionals; in fact, the process should encourage the family to be their own advocates. Underlying the supposition of enabling and empowering the family are three assumptions: (1) the family is competent or is capable of being competent, (2) enablement and empowerment create opportunities for the family to exhibit their competence, and (3) empowerment creates opportunities for meeting family concerns in ways that promote the family's control over their lives and that of the infant or toddler (Dunst, Trivette, & Deal, 1988; Espe-Sherwindt & Kerlin, 1990).

Based on Family Concerns

An effective assessment is based on concerns as specified by the family. Winton (1996) indicates that if an assessment is to be family centered, the "first order of business is to find out what families want" (p. 31). The desired outcomes for intervention should be those that the family has identified. When family goals and objectives were obtained from caregivers and incorporated into the child's individualized family service plan (IFSP), the result consisted of goals that were more "functional, generic, easy to integrate within the instructional context and measurable" (Notari & Drinkwater, 1991, p. 100).

Coordinated with Other Community Agencies

An effective assessment views the child and the family in a larger circle that incorporates other services that a family may receive. The federal legislation requires that there be coordination of the early intervention services and other services that the child needs or is being provided. Thus the service coordinator and the early intervention program administrators work with the family to coordinate services from traditional intervention services such as education, special education, allied health services, and daycare, to more diverse services that the family may need, such as public social services, health services, Medicaid, health maintenance organization or insurance reimbursement, and parent support and advocacy groups.

Normalized

Effective assessments are normalized. Assessment is based on natural observation of the child's communicative abilities in the context of naturally occurring routines and events. Therefore when planning and subsequently completing this assessment, care must be taken when choosing the location in which the assessment will be completed. Will the assessment be completed in the child's home, at a school or agency, or at a neutral site? For an assessment to be normalized, care should be taken not only in determining the location of the assessment but also in determining what time of day the assessment is to be completed. It is ideal for the assessment to occur at a time that "allows maximum participation by the child's caregiver and within a context that promotes typical interaction with the child" (Crais, 1996, p. 73). For example, it does not make sense to assess an infant's or toddler's feeding abilities after he or she has eaten if your goal is to observe the child during this normally occurring event.

Involving Professionals from Other Disciplines

P.L. 99-457 requires that an assessment of handicapped infants, toddlers, and preschoolers be conducted by a multi-disciplinary team; therefore an effective assessment involves other professionals. Team members are expected to represent their disciplines and report their findings to other members of the team, including the family (or its representative) (Fewell, 1991). The multi-disciplinary team, in partnership with the family, develops the assessment outcomes and the IFSP. This team may include the child and the family, the service coordinator, and various professionals such as the speech–language pathologist, audiologist, educators, physical and occupational therapists, physicians, other heath care providers, daycare staff, and social workers.

Comprehensive

Effective assessment is comprehensive, covering all the important developmental and behavioral dimensions of language and communication, and considers the child's performance across natural settings. At the very least, the communication assessment must consider the child's comprehension of language, expression of intentionality and the form of such communication, ability to engage in interactions with supportive partners, and language-related cognitive abilities (Crais, 1995; Prizant & Wetherby, 1993). New York State recommends that an in-depth speech–language evaluation include the following: (1) assessment of hearing ability and hearing history, (2) history of speech–language development, (3) oral motor functioning and feeding history, (4) expressive and receptive language performance, (5) social development, (6) quality/resonance of voice, and (7) fluency (Clinical Practice Guideline, 1999, p. III-69).

ASSESSMENT OUTCOMES

The outcome of an assessment that follows the guidelines presented for an effective assessment will be one that not only identifies the family's concerns about the child's communication abilities but also, in so doing, identifies the goals of intervention. Goals of an effective assessment may include the following:

- To identify family concerns, priorities, and resources.
- To identify the infant's or toddler's strengths and needs.
- To identify the focus of intervention as well as ecologically valid contexts for intervention.
- To develop consensus on family concerns, priorities and resources, infant's strengths and needs, focus of intervention, and valid intervention contexts.
- To reinforce parents' feelings of competence and worth.
- To develop ownership of decisions and plans by all parties involved.

Before a discussion of the different outcomes of an effective assessment in harmony with our family-centered approach can occur, it must be realized that reports should be written so as to "take into account the language, culture, and literacy level of the intended readers" (Miller & Hanft, 1998, p. 56). It should be remembered that the report is written for both parents and other professionals. In addition, "information about test scores or a diagnosis should be provided with explanations. Fact and opinion should be clearly distinguished and all available opinions presented" (Berman & Shaw, 1996, p. 370).

Identification of Family Concerns

Family concerns, priorities, and resources can be identified in a variety of ways, but probably the most effective way is to ask the family what they are. The early interventionist should remember that the focus is not to evaluate families but to ascertain what the family hopes to accomplish through the assessment and the early intervention process. Many tools and strategies have been reported in the literature to accomplish this task (Winton, 1996). One practical strategy for gathering family information is the use of a traditional set of questions (oral or written) designed to elicit this information. The information gathered usually concerns the child's medical, prenatal, birth, and developmental history as well as family background and demographic information. Winton (1996) indicates that although this may be a method for obtaining standardized information about all children and families, some families perceive this "as being intrusive and perhaps violating their right to privacy" (p. 45). Another method of obtaining information related to family concerns, priorities, and resources is the use of a self-report questionnaire such as the *Family Needs Survey* (Bailey & Simeonsson, 1985). Bailey and Blascoe (1990) report that families indicate that they do not consider such a questionnaire to be intrusive. A third means of obtaining family information is through informal interviews. Summers, Dell'Oliver, Turnbull, Benson, Santelli, Campbell & Siegal-Causey (1990) suggest that parents prefer informal interviews to a more standardized formal questionnaire.

Identification of Infant-Toddler Strengths and Needs

To identify the infant's or toddler's strengths and needs the interventionist must plan and complete an assessment. Assessments should focus on the infant's or toddler's strengths and abilities, what he or she can communicate, and the manner in which this is accomplished. A comprehensive description of the child's strengths and abilities must be the result of such an assessment so that the family can gain insight into the child's needs.

Identification of Focus of Intervention and Ecologically Valid Contexts for Intervention

Another outcome of such an assessment is the determination of areas the family designates for intervention, as well as a determination of ecologically valid contexts for intervention or the naturally occurring routines in which communication takes place. When establishing the contexts for intervention, Wetherby and Prizant (1996) indicate that two aspects of the communication environment must be considered: the quality and quantity of opportunities for communicating, and the interaction strategies used by communicative partners (p. 307).

Developing Consensus

In a family-centered assessment, the parents or caregivers identify their issues and concerns for the child, as does the professional. The collaboration between the family and the professional results in prioritization of the desired outcomes. The purpose of prioritizing is not to reduce the number of goals but rather to ensure that those factors that are highly valued by the family are addressed by the intervention plan (McWilliam, 1996, p. 106).

Reinforcing Parents' Feelings of Competence and Worth

Crais (1994) indicates that when we incorporate families into the assessment process we should reinforce parents' feelings of competence and worth. Sometimes families with infants and toddlers in need of early intervention services feel incapable of caring for their young child, or sometimes professionals inadvertently make the family feel less competent.

Developing Ownership of Decisions and Plans by All Parties Involved

Assessment should be a collaborative process between professionals and families striving to build an understanding of the child in the context of his or her family. If the assessment is collaborative, all parties involved will feel ownership of the outcomes and intervention plan (Crais, 1994). If all parties feel this ownership, they can work together to facilitate the infant or toddler's development.

SUMMARY OF ASSESSMENT OUTCOMES

The assessment process previously described is different from a traditional assessment of a young child, which is conducted by the professional and relies on results of formal testing under standard conditions (Crais, 1994). The results of the formal testing procedures in turn result in a diagnostic label. Professionals may share results with other professionals and in turn develop recommendations made by professionals without family input. This is a professionally driven model of assessment (Crais, 1994). This traditional model has numerous limitations due to lack of involvement of the caregivers. It promotes the notion of professional expertise, whereas it is apparent that professionals in a one-hour visit cannot know the child as well as the caregivers who spend considerable time with the infant or toddler. By promoting professional expertise, professionals are sustaining a belief of parental incompetence (Crais, 1994). Thus caregivers feel "disenfranchised" from the assessment process and may not commit to the professionally driven model. Disenfranchisement is a consequence of lack of consensus concerning desired outcomes. When caregivers are disenfranchised, they do not commit to the professionally developed programming, resulting in discontinuity of programming for the child or minimal follow-through by caregivers.

If an assessment generally follows the assumptions previously discussed, both professionals and families assume a variety of roles. These roles are enacted after multiple means of obtaining information are determined. The choice of assessment tools and techniques may be based on many considerations. These may include the following:

- The family's desired outcome for the assessment, with an eye to the family's needs, resources, priorities, strengths, and supports.
- The family's preference for how the assessment occurs, with a focus on multiple opportunities for the family to provide input.
- Matching the family's background, culture, language, or any combination of these.
- Professional's goals for the assessment.
- Areas of concern and areas of strength (characteristics of the child).
- Context in which the assessment takes place, with an eye to incorporating the family environment.
- Time or other constraints.

MEANS OF ASSESSMENT

Assessments should involve multiple sources of information and multiple components. Greenspan and Meisels (1996) indicate that an assessment should include a variety of information from a variety of perspectives. When adapting their perspective to communication assessment (which is a focused observation of a specific area of the child's functioning) the following should be included: (1) the parents' description of the child's capacities, (2) the parents' detailed descriptions of the child's developmental history, (3) direct observation of the child, including interaction between the child and the caregiver, and (4) a description of the child's functional communication capabilities.

To obtain this information, there are at least three means of assessment, which include (1) parent interview, report, and participation, (2) formal or structured methods or both, and (3) informal observations.

Parent Interview, Report, and Participation

Parent interviews and reports are a useful means of obtaining information. Typically, interviews are used to obtain information about parental concern and background as well as developmental information. Use of parental concerns as the determining factor when deciding if an infant or toddler is in need of intervention has been effective (Diamond, 1987; Diamond, 1993). In a family-centered assessment, interviewing is a tool that the professional may use to obtain information about the family's concerns and the child's strengths. The professional needs to adapt his or her interviewing skills to be family focused. Many suggest (Andrews & Andrews, 1995; Briggs, 1998; Winton, 1996) that an initial open-ended question allows the family to best express their issues. At this time, the role of the professional is to sit patiently and silently to allow the family's story to unfold (Briggs, 1998). Winton (1996) indicates that there are four skills that professionals should possess when collaborating with families. These include listening, reflecting feelings, reflecting content, and questioning effectively (p. 51). To listen effectively, the professional should attend to what family members have to say using both verbal and nonverbal listening skills. Briggs (1998) stresses the importance of using focused listening (listening and integrating what the family says) rather than jumping to the next question when interviewing families. Therefore the professional needs to know how to use questions to their fullest, as well as when to remain silent and listen. Winton (1996) states that reflecting feelings includes "perceiving accurately and sensitively the feelings of family members and communicating that understanding in appropriate language" (p. 51). Andrews (1986) includes these skills when she says that professionals need to be nonjudgmental in order to really listen to the family. Another skill that Winton (1996) considers important in working with families is the ability to restate the content of discussions with families by reiterating and summarizing the family's messages. When reflecting the content of family discussions it is important to accept differing points of views (Andrews, 1986). Briggs (1998) recommends that professionals learn to use mirroring, which involves reflecting the tone, mannerism, language, affect, and style of the family in order to build a trusting relationship.

Another important aspect in gathering background information from caregivers and families is that the early interventionist must be culturally sensitive. Barrera (1996) indicates that there are three dimensions of the socio-cultural context that should be taken into consideration when assessing the needs and the strengths of young children and their families. These include the personal–social dimension, the communicative–linguistic dimension, and the sensory–cognitive dimension (p. 75). See Table 2-1 for the types of information that would be included in each of the three dimensions of the socio-cultural context.

Another focus of interviews stems from the realization that parents and caregivers in their daily observations have a wealth of information about their children doing things in contexts that interventionists cannot observe, and

Table 2-1	*Three dimensions of the sociocultural context*
DIMENSION	**CHARACTERISTICS**
Personal-Social	Includes – the child or family's degree of acculturation – the child's personal-social knowledge and skills – the child or family's sense of identity
Communicative-Linguistic	Includes – family or community's value and type(s) of communication – child's language proficiency—both (all) languages – disparity between the language of the home environment and the early intervention environment (includes complexity of language used, topic of conversation, and use of verbal/nonverbal language) – language and sense of self; includes which language the family feels more comfortable expressing affect
Sensory-Cognitive	Includes – comfort, preference, and value of learning styles of home and the child – disparity between the home and early intervention environment's categories of knowledge: what is valued and what is promoted – family's belief of the value and role of early intervention

Adapted from Barrera, I. (1996). Thoughts on the assessment of young children whose sociocultural background is unfamiliar to the assessor. In Meisels, S. & Fenichel, E. M. (Eds.) *New visions for the assessment of infants and young children* pp. 69-84. Washington, D.C.: Zero to Three.

that this information provides an accurate picture of the infant or toddler. To assess the communicative competence of an infant or toddler, it is important to obtain information about his or her home ecology. Even if the assessment team makes a home visit, in a limited time frame it is not possible to fully observe an infant's or toddler's communicative abilities. It should be remembered that an infant's or toddler's communication is highly dependent on the context. Thus assessment is based on observations in all of the child's contexts to allow the interventionist to develop a complete picture of the child's abilities. Since this is not a possibility for professionals, interviewing the caregivers about the child's abilities in all environments provides the necessary information. The literature provides examples of interviews that are focused on specific areas of communication and procedures for completing these interviews. For example, Schuler, Peck, Willard, and Theimer (1989) present a format for interviewing caregivers about a child's expression of communicative intent (why the child communicates), and Rescorla (1989) presents a format for collecting information about the size of a child's vocabulary. Thus caregivers can provide the interventionist with valuable information about the unique characteristics of the infant or toddler, which can facilitate the professionals' interaction with the child. Roberts and Crais (1989) provide a format for using interviews as a means of obtaining information about the communicative intentions the child is currently expressing, the mode of the communicative attempts (words or gestures), and the situations in which the child expresses the communicative intents.

Some informal questions that focus more specifically on communicative abilities are as follows:

- How does the child express needs (e.g., hunger, thirst, desire for something, emotions)? (If needed, offer gestures, words, vocalizations, and so forth)
- How does the child react when his or her needs are met or not met?
- How do others understand the child's communicative attempts? How does the child express needs to others?
- How does the child participate in family routines (e.g., dinner time, bath time)?
- How does the child respond when spoken to?
- Who does the child interact with most often?

Additional informal questions that focus more specifically on socialization and play may include the following:

- What activities does the child enjoy?
- What are the child's favorite games and toys? What does the child do with these toys?
- Who does the child play with?
- What does the child enjoy?
- What upsets the child?

In addition, when working with families from diverse cultural backgrounds, interviews may or may not be an excellent means of obtaining information about the child. For some families, an interview singles out the child and the family; in other families, interviews on sensitive topics (e.g., questions related to marital relationships) are inappropriate and thus culturally insensitive. The role of the professional in gathering interview data is to "determine when and how data gathering and assessment can be conducted in a culturally competent manner" (Lynch & Hanson, 1998, p. 503).

The literature (Dale, Bates, Reznick, & Morisset, 1989; Rescorla, 1989; Reznick & Goldsmith, 1989) strongly supports parental reporting techniques as a valid and effective way of measuring language development. The information obtained from a formal parent report instrument has been used as the primary means of making a decision if a referral is needed in screenings (Bricker & Squires, 1989; Diamond & Squires, 1993), in addition to being one piece of a total assessment. Diamond and Squires (1993) present five guidelines for increasing the agreement between professional and family assessment. As reported by Diamond and Squires (1993), these include: (1) targeting current observable behaviors, (2) focusing on frequently occurring behaviors, (3) using a recognition format rather than a recall format, (4) establishing parent skill level to be at a level needed to complete the questionnaire or interview, and (5) providing an opportunity to parents to observe their child rather than to speculate on behavior (p. 112).

An example of a parent report measure that uses a recognition format is the *MacArthur Communicative Development Inventories (CDI)* (Fenson et al., 1993). The *CDI* protocol consists of two parts. Part I is a vocabulary checklist, which requires the primary caregiver to indicate which words he or she believes the child uses expressively or understands. Part II obtains information regarding sentence use, grammar, and complexity of the child's language use. A more traditional instrument that uses a parent report format is the *Receptive Expressive Emergent Language Scale III* (Bzoch, League & Brown, 2003). This assessment instrument is a language development checklist that can be completed through parent report or professional observation. In addition, other assessment instruments use parent report as one of many means of determining if a specific child behavior is present. One example is the *Rossetti Infant Toddler Language Scale* (Rossetti, 1990).

Formal and Structured Assessment Methods

Formal means of assessment include a variety of standardized tests, criterion-referenced measures, and structured observational procedures. Many of these formal assessment methods rely on observation-based methodologies. These assessment tools are "the most formal, decontextualized format for assessing language function. They are developed by devising a series of items that are then given to (ideally) large groups of normal children and computing the acceptable range of variation in scores for the age range covered by the test" (Paul, 2001, p. 38). During assessment of young children, the child's achievement of developmental milestones typically serves as the basis for these assessment instruments. These developmentally based instruments can either be highly structured or serve as informal checklists for the interventionists. When using a formal test instrument to determine if the infant or toddler is eligible for services, the interventionist should be aware that the same test instrument may not be appropriate for determining the infant's or toddler's strengths and needs. There are a variety of reasons why early interventionists may decide to use a formal test instrument. Some of these reasons reflect the positive characteristics of these instruments, yet the early interventionist must be careful when using these more formal instruments, as there are some inherent concerns.

First, the positive characteristics of formal assessment instruments should be considered. The results of a formal assessment procedure can allow the professional to make comparisons between the child being assessed and other children at the same age or developmental level. Other positive characteristics of formal assessment instruments include the fact that (1) they are accompanied by normative data that can be used to quantify a child's current developmental level and (2) they can be used to identify children with disabilities. In addition, formal assessment instruments have clear administration and scoring criteria, which makes them relatively easy to administer, and many have established protocols and sets of materials. Some formal assessment instruments can measure general change over time (Crais, 1995; Weitzner-Lin, 1994). In addition, formal assessment tools have documented reliability and validity, and they may be used for program planning. Even though there are many positive characteristics of formal assessment instruments, the professional needs to be aware of weaknesses as well. Limitations that reflect professional dissatisfaction with formal tools include the following:

- Formal tools are not designed to guide intervention planning, and the information obtained about the infant or toddler does not specify what strategies to use with that child when providing intervention.
- Formal tools provide a limited view of the child's communication skills in naturalistic contexts.
- Formal tests typically target the form of communication (gestures, words, and multiword combinations) rather than looking at communication from a larger interactive perspective (looking at communicative functions expressed, as well as the success of these communicative attempts in real interactions).
- Formal tests do not typically use caregivers as active participants in the interactive process or in the assessment process as a whole.
- A composite view of the child's overall skills is not available when test items are administered, as they do not represent a global view of the child's communication skills. In other words, there is no specific indication of how the child is actually communicating.
- Formal tests do not provide a profile of early communicative behavior (preverbal communication, communicative functions, social–affective components, spontaneous initiation); rather, they focus on what the child cannot do without elaborating on what he or she can do, or they give a global view of the child.
- Most formal tests allow for minimal adaptations to match the child's characteristics. Since many infants or toddlers are too young to cooperate with a structured format, many formal measures are difficult to administer.
- Formal tests tend to be clinician driven, which limits the opportunity to observe and document spontaneous communication abilities.
- Despite the existence of an established protocol and set of materials, a formal test may be difficult to administer to a young child because of the lack of contextual support for the child, as well as the child's limited experiences with standardized testing procedures.
- Formal assessment instruments are not culturally sensitive.

As practicing early interventionists, it is important to ask if the test properly samples the prelinguistic and early linguistic behaviors basic to communicative development. Wetherby and Prizant (1992) and Crais (1995) have reviewed many of the formal speech and language assessment instruments from such a framework and have indicated that these instruments do not comprehensively assess all developmental and behavioral dimensions of communicative abilities.

Crais (1995) analyzed frequently administered formal assessment tools on a set of 13 characteristics that are part of an effective assessment. Crais found that most of the formal assessment tools and techniques address several of the characteristics and that when the formal test instruments typically do not focus on some aspect, they can be adapted to address it. However, the professional should remember that this presents a "catch-22" for the assessor because once a formal standardized assessment instrument is adapted, it no longer provides the professional with valid scores or results.

If a formal assessment instrument is to be administered, the selection of such an instrument should be based on that instrument's completeness with regard to the goals of the assessment. However, as Wetherby and Prizant (1992) indicate, there are currently no formal measures of communication that assess early communication behaviors in a systematic and comprehensive manner. Thus the speech–language early interventionist finds it necessary to augment standardized tests with less formal and more observational techniques to gain a more representative picture of the child's communication skills.

Informal Approaches and Observations

Observation in early assessment is considered a critical aspect of a complete assessment because the observation may provide information about the way in which the infant or toddler uses his or her communication skills to achieve real communicative outcomes. It has been recognized for some time now that informal observation in a comfortable setting may be more important for the speech–language evaluation than the use of a standardized assessment tool (McCune, Kalmanson, Fleck, Glazewski, & Sillari, 1990; Weitzner-Lin, 1994). The context in which these observations occur is critical because they will impact the infant's or toddler's communication. Much of a prelinguistic and early linguistic child's communication is context bound in that the intended message can only be derived from the context in which the message is issued. Children display their communicative abilities through gestures, which can only be interpreted in the context in which they are used. The early interventionist must be careful when deciding on the context to observe because of the influence of the context on early communication. Here again, caregivers have a vital role in the assessment process because they are the best source of determining which context is most fruitful for communication. Home-based observation probably allows for more comfort and freedom on the part of both the child and the caregiver, and thus provides a richer sample of the child's communicative abilities.

In addition to paying attention to the context in which the communication sample is collected, the early interventionist should remember that other aspects of the interaction could affect the representativeness of the sample collected. Interactant variables also have an impact on the sample. The most natural interactive partner for a young child is his or her caregiver. Ideally, a communication sample can be obtained between the caregiver and the child, as it is with the caregiver that the child will most probably demonstrate his or her typical communication patterns. If the early interventionist must be the interactive partner, he or she must "listen, be patient, follow the child's lead, not ask dumb questions, and consider the child's perspective" (Miller, 1981, as cited in Paul, 2001, p. 47).

Another concern about observation is whether observation is enough. In other words, can a true picture of a child's communicative performance be obtained through observation alone? Investigators (Coggins, Olswang & Guthrie, 1987; Wetherby & Rodriguez, 1992) have found that natural contexts are good for sampling some types of communicative behavior (e.g., expression of comments), whereas other types of assessment (structured elicitation) were better for other behaviors (sampling expression of requests). Thus researchers (Coggins et al., 1987; Wetherby & Rodriguez, 1992) believe that observation alone will not tap into an infant or toddler's true communicative performance, as it does not obtain information about all types of communicative functions.

The limitations of low-structured observations to obtain information about all communicative functions appear to be related to the characteristics of the situation, particularly the impact of the play materials on the type of communication expressed. Holdgrafter and Dunst (1990) suggest that the early interventionist carefully arrange the communicative situation to obtain information about the child's ability to comment and request primarily in reference to the immediate context, or to communicate about displaced topics (prompted by objects in the immediate situation or based totally on mental representation). Contextual variables play an important part in the observation of the young child. The context might not be supportive of a particular type of communication, time constraints may limit the amount of communication sampled, the naturalness of context may still be contrived, the communicative partner may be inhibited because of the observer, and, of course, the stimulus materials may affect what topics are discussed and the types of communicative intents that can be expressed. Holdgrafer and Dunst (1990) suggest that to use low-structured observations to their fullest, the clinician (examiner, parent) should carefully determine what information is needed and the appropriate characteristics of the event in which the observation will occur.

To overcome the limitations previously discussed, the interventionist should use elicitation tasks (and parent report) to augment the observations. Elicitation tasks (sometimes called communication temptations) do not guarantee that a specific behavior will be sampled, but they increase the likelihood that the young child will produce the desired behavior in a given situation. The types of elicitation tasks that are discussed in the literature are elicited imitation and elicited production. Elicited imitation can best be described as the assessor asking the child to "say what I say and do what I do." Lund and Duchan (1993) indicate that this form of elicitation is pragmatically flawed in the sense that in real conversation we do not usually repeat what the other person has said. Elicited production is pragmatically more appropriate in that the assessor tempts the child to express a particular thing by setting up the context. The context encourages the child to produce a specific utterance appropriate to that context. Wetherby and Prizant (1989) have developed a series of "communication temptations" to elicit the expression of intentional communicative utterances by young children. They indicate that these elicitation procedures are useful for the child who does not initiate freely. These authors indicate that the use of "communicative temptations involves creating opportunities that entice specific attempts at communication, that they are appropriate for children functioning between the prelinguistic and two-word stage and can be easily modified and tailored for each individual child" (p. 85). See Box 2-2 for a description of the communicative temptations suggested by Wetherby and Prizant (1989).

Box 2-2	*Communicative temptations*

- Eat a desired food item in front of the child without offering any to the child.
- Activate a wind-up toy, let it deactivate, and hand it to the child.
- Give the child four blocks to drop in a box, one at a time (or use some other action that the child will repeat, such as stacking the blocks or dropping the blocks on the floor); then immediately give the child a small animal figure to drop in the box.
- Look through a few books or a magazine with the child.
- Open a jar of bubbles, blow bubbles, and then close the jar tightly and give the closed jar to the child.
- Initiate a familiar and an unfamiliar social game with the child until the child expresses pleasure, then stop the game and wait.
- Blow up a balloon and slowly deflate it, then hand the deflated balloon to the child or hold the deflated balloon up to your mouth and wait.
- Hold a food item or toy that the child dislikes out near the child to offer it.
- Place a desired food item or toy in a clear container that the child cannot open while the child is watching; then put the container in front of the child and wait.
- Place the child's hands in a cold, wet, or sticky substance, such as Jello, pudding, or paste.
- Roll a ball to the child; after the child returns the ball three times, immediately roll a different toy to the child.
- Engage the child in putting together a puzzle. After the child has put in three pieces, offer the child a piece that does not fit.
- Engage the child in an activity with a substance that can be easily spilled (or dropped, broken, torn, etc.); suddenly spill some of the substance on the table or floor in front of the child and wait.
- Put an object that makes noise in an opaque container and shake it; hold up the container and wait.
- Give the child the materials for an activity of interest that necessitates the use of an instrument for completion (e.g., piece of paper to draw on or cut; bowl of pudding or soup), hold the instrument out of the child's reach and wait.
- Engage the child in an activity of interest that necessitates the use of an instrument for completion (e.g., pen, crayon, scissors, stapler, wand for blowing bubbles, spoon), have a third person come over and take the instrument, go sit on the distant side of the room while holding the instrument within the child's sight, and wait.
- Wave and say "bye" to an object upon removing it from the play area. Repeat this for a second and third situation, and do nothing when removing an object from the fourth situation. These four trials should be presented following four consecutive temptations above.
- Hide a stuffed animal under the table. Knock, and then bring out the animal. Have the animal greet the child the first time. Repeat this for a second and third time, and do nothing when bringing out the animal the fourth time. These four trials should also be interspersed with the temptations above when presented.

From Wetherby, A., & Prizant, B. (1989). The expression of communicative intent: Assessment guidelines. *Seminars in Speech and Language, 10*(1):77-91.

SUMMARY OF MEANS OF ASSESSMENT

The discussion concerning observation and elicitation tasks reminds us that multiple measures and multiple sources of information are needed for an effective assessment. These multiple sources of information should be completed across multiple occasions because the young child's attention and stamina may be challenged. The speech–language early interventionist should remember that if a particular linguistic ability is not sampled in a particular context, it does not mean that the behavior is not part of the child's repertoire. It may mean that contextual variables and evaluator characteristics are the real concerns. The communicative assessment should thus take place in an interactive and meaningful context where the child's caregiver is completely involved. Thus a more complete assessment will include samples of spontaneous communication obtained in natural contexts, observations of communication in natural contexts, structured elicitation, parent report, and sometimes the results of standardized expressive or receptive language tests.

REFERENCES

Andrews, M. A. (1986). Application of family therapy techniques to the treatment of language disorders. *Seminars in Speech and Language, 7*(4), 347-358.

Andrews, J. R., & Andrews, M. A. (1995). Solution-focused assumptions that support family-centered early intervention. *Infants and Young Children,* 8(1), 60-67.

Bailey, D. B., & Blascoe, P. (1990). Parents' perspective on a written survey of family needs. *Journal of Early Intervention,* 14(3), 196-203.

Bailey, D. B., & Simeonsson, R. J. (1985). *Family needs scale.* Chapel Hill, NC: Frank Porter Graham Child Development Center, University of North Carolina.

Barrera, I. (1996). Thoughts on the assessment of young children whose sociocultural background is unfamiliar to the assessor. In S. Meisels & E. M. Fenichel (Eds.), *New visions for the assessment of infants and young children* (pp. 69-84). Washington, DC: Zero to Three.

Battle, D. E. (1997). Language and communication disorders in culturally and linguistically diverse children. In D. K. Bernstein & E. Tiegerman-Farber (Eds.), *Language and communication disorders in children* (4th Ed.) (pp. 382-409). Boston: Allyn & Bacon.

Berman, C., & Shaw, E. (1996). Family-directed child evaluation and assessment under the individuals with disabilities education act (IDEA). In S. J. Meisels & E. Fenichel (Eds.), *New visions for the developmental assessment of infants and young children* (pp. 361-390). Washington DC: Zero to Three.

Bricker, D., & Squires, J. (1989). The effectiveness of screening of at-risk infants: Infant Monitoring Questionnaires. *Topics in Early Childhood Special Education, 9*(3), 67-85.

Briggs, M. H. (1998). Families talk: Building partnerships for communicative change. *Topics in Language Disorders,* 18(3), 71-84.

Bzoch, K. R., League, R. & Brown, V. (2003). *Receptive expressive emergent language scale–III* (3rd Ed.) TX: ProEd.

Chan, S. (1990). Early intervention with culturally diverse families of infants and toddlers with disabilities. *Infants and Young Children,* 3(2), 78-87.

Clinical practice guideline: The guideline technical report. *Communication disorders, assessment and intervention for young children (age 0–3 years)* (1999). Albany, NY: New York State Department of Health, Early Intervention Program.

Coggins, T. E., Olswang, L. B., & Guthrie, J. (1987). Assessing communicative intents in young children: Low structured observation or elicitation tasks. *Journal of Speech and Hearing Disorders, 52*, 44-49.

Crais, E. R. (1996). Applying family-centered principles to child assessment. In P. J. William, P. J. Winton, & E. R. Crais (Eds.), *Practical strategies for family-centered intervention* (pp. 69-96). San Diego: Singular Publishing Group.

Crais, E. R. (1995). Expanding the repertoire of tools and techniques for assessing communication skills of infants and toddlers. *American Journal of Speech–Language Pathology, 4*(3), 47-59.

Crais, E. R. (1994). *Increasing family participation: In the assessment of children birth to five.* Itasca, IL: Riverside Publishing Company.

Dale, P.S., Bates, E., Reznick, J.S., & Morisset, C. (1989). The validity of a parent report instrument of child language at 20 months. *Journal of Child Language, 16*, 239-249.

Diamond, K. (1987). Predicting school problems from preschool development screening: A four-year follow-up of the Revised Denver Developmental Screening Test and the role of parent report. *Journal of the Division for Early Childhood, 11*, 247-253.

Diamond, K. E. (1993). The role of parents' observations and concerns in screening for developmental delays in young children. *Topics in Early Childhood Special Education, 13*(1), 68-81.

Diamond, K., & Squires, J. (1993). The role of parental report in screening and assessment of young children. *Journal of Early Intervention, 17*(2), 107-115.

Dunst C. J., Trivette, C. M., & Deal, A. G. (1988). *Enabling and empowering families: Principles and guidelines for practice.* Cambridge, MA: Brookline Books.

Eiserman, W. D., Weber, C., & McCoun, M. (1995). Parent and professional roles in early intervention: A longitudinal comparison of the effects of two intervention configurations. *The Journal of Special Education, 29*(1), 20-44.

Espe-Sherwindt, M., & Kerlin, S. L. (1990). Early intervention with parents with mental retardation: Do we empower or impair? *Infants and Young Children, 2*(4), 21-28.

Fenson, L., Dale, P. S., Reznick, J. S., Thal, D., Bates, E., Hartung, J. P., Pethick, S., & Reilly, J. (1993). *MacArthur communicative development inventories: User's guide and technical manual.* San Diego: Singular Publishing Group.

Fewell, R. R. (1991). Trends in the assessment of infants and toddlers with disabilities. *Exceptional Children,* (October-November), 166-173.

Greenspan, S. I., & Meisels, S. J. (1996). Toward a new vision of developmental assessment of infants and young children. In S. J. Meisels & E. Fenichel (Eds.), *New visions for the developmental assessment of infants and young children* (pp. 11-26). Washington, DC: Zero to Three.

Henderson, L. W., & Meisels, S. J. (1994). Parental involvement in the developmental screening of their young children: Multiple-source perspective. *Journal of Early Intervention, 18*(2), 141-154.

Holdgrafer, G. E., & Dunst, C. J. (1990). Use of low structured observation for assessing communicative intents in young children. *First Language, 10*, 243-253.

Leviton, A., Mueller, M., & Kauffman, C. (1992). The family-centered consultation model: Practical applications for professionals. *Infants and Young Children, 4*(3), 1-8.

Lund, N.J. & Duchan, J.F. (1993). *Assessing children's language in naturalistic contexts* (3rd ed.). Englewood Cliffs, NJ: Prentice Hall.

Lynch, E. W., & Hanson, M. J. (1998). Steps in the right direction: Implications for interventionists. In Lynch, E. W. & Hanson, M. J. (Eds.), *Developing cross-cultural competence: A guide for working with children and their families* (2nd ed) (pp. 491-512). Baltimore, MD: Paul H. Brooks Publishing Co.

McCune, L., Kalmanson, B., Fleck, M.B., Glazewski, B., & Sillari, J. (1990). An interdisciplinary model of infant assessment. In S. J. Meisels & J. P. Shonkoff (Eds.), *Handbook of early childhood intervention* (pp. 219-245). New York: Cambridge University Press.

McWilliam, P. J. (1996). Family-centered intervention planning. In P. J. McWilliam, P. J. Winton, & E.R. Crais (Eds.), *Practical strategies for family-centered intervention* (pp. 97-123). San Diego: Singular Publishing Group.

Miller, L. J., & Hanft, B. E. (1998). Building positive alliances: Partnerships with families as the cornerstone of developmental assessment. *Infants and Young Children, 11*(1), 49-60.

Notari, A. R., & Drinkwater, S. G. (1991). Best practices for writing child outcomes: An evaluation of two methods. *Topics in Early Childhood Special Education, 11*(3), 92-106.

Paul, R. (2001). *Language disorders from infancy through adolescence: Assessment and intervention* (2nd ed.). St. Louis, MO: Mosby.

Prizant, B., & Wetherby, A. (1993). Communication and language assessment for young children. *Infants and Young Children, 5*(4), 20-34.

Rescorla, L. (1989). The language development survey: A screening tool for delayed language in toddlers. *Journal of Speech and Hearing Disorders, 54*, 587-599.

Reznick, J. S., & Goldsmith, L. (1989). A multiple form word production checklist for assessing early language. *Journal of Child Language, 16*, 91-100.

Richard, N. B., & Schiefelbusch, R. L. (1990). Assessment. In L. McCormick & R. L. Schiefelbusch (Eds.), *Early language intervention: An introduction* (2nd ed.). Columbus, OH: Merrill Publishing Co.

Roberts, J. E., & Crais, E. R. (1989). Assessing communication skills. In D. B. Bailey & M. Wolery (Eds.), *Assessing infants and preschoolers with handicaps* (pp. 339-389). Columbus, OH: Merrill Publishing Co.

Rossetti, L. (1990). *Infant Toddler Language Scale.* East Moline, IL: Lingua Systems Inc.

Schuler, A. L., Peck, C. A., Willard, C., & Theimer, K. (1989). Assessment of communicative means and functions through interview: Assessing the communicative abilities of individuals with limited language. *Seminars in Speech and Language, 10*, 51-62.

Summers, J. A., Dell'Oliver, C., Turnbull, A. P., Benson, H. A., Santelli, E., Campbell, M., & Siegal-Causey, E. (1990). Examining the individualized family service plan process: What are family and practitioner preferences? *Topics in Early Childhood Special Education, 10*(1), 78-99.

Weitzner-Lin, B. (1994). Communication and language. In J. Bonderant-Utz & L. Luciano (Eds.), *A practical guide to infant and preschool assessment in special education* (pp. 241-261). Boston: Allyn & Bacon.

Weitzner-Lin, B. (1992). Infants and toddlers: Contemporary assessment issues. Weitzner-Lin, B. and Crais, E. Infants and Toddlers. Miniseminar. New York State Speech Language and Hearing Association. Kiamesha Lake, NY, April.

Wetherby, A. M., & Prizant, B. M. (1996). Toward earlier identification of communication and language problems in infants and young children. In S. J. Meisels & E. Fenichel (Eds.), *New visions for the developmental assessment of infants and young children* (pp. 289-312). Washington, DC: Zero to Three.

Wetherby, A. M., & Prizant, B. M. (1992). Profiling young children's communicative competence. In S. Warren & J. Reichle (Eds.), *Causes and effects in communication and language intervention* (pp. 217-251). Baltimore, MD: Paul H. Brookes Publishing Co.

Wetherby, A. M., & Prizant, B. M. (1989). The expression of communicative intent: Assessment guidelines. *Seminars in Speech and Language, 10*(1), 77-91.

Wetherby, A. M., & Rodriguez, G. P. (1992). Measurement of communicative intentions. *Journal of Speech and Hearing Research, 35*, 130-138.

Winton, P. J. (1996). Understanding family concerns, priorities and resources. In P. J. William, P. J. Winton, & E. R. Crais (Eds.), *Practical strategies for family-centered intervention* (pp. 31-53). San Diego: Singular Publishing Group.

C H A P T E R   3

Components of a Speech-Language-Communication Assessment

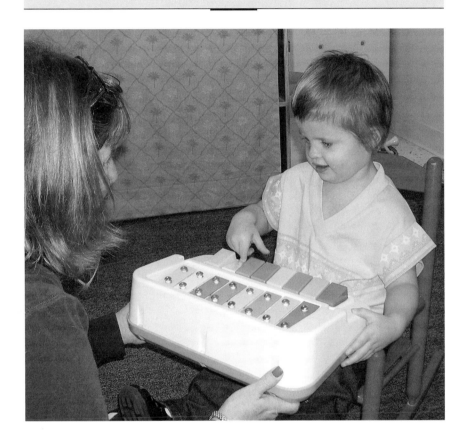

OUTLINE

INTENTIONALITY
HOW TO ASSESS INTENTIONALITY
PHONOLOGY
HOW TO ASSESS PHONOLOGY
VERBAL FORM
ALTERNATIVE MODES OF
  COMMUNICATION
PLAY
HOW TO DO A PLAY ASSESSMENT AND
  WHAT TO LOOK FOR

CAREGIVER–CHILD INTERACTION:
  CAREGIVER VARIABLES
CAREGIVER–CHILD INTERACTION:
  CHILD VARIABLES
LANGUAGE COMPREHENSION
ORAL–MOTOR ABILITIES
AUDIOLOGICAL EVALUATION
SUMMARY

This chapter presents a detailed discussion of the components of a comprehensive communication assessment. Beginning with the concept that an infant must have something to communicate (an intent) and a form in which to transmit that intent, the chapter further elaborates on (1) the role of parent or caregiver–child interaction in communication development, (2) play as a means of assessing knowledge that underlies communication, (3) comprehension, and (4) other sensory and motor components of communication (audition, oral motor skills, and so forth).

A detailed discussion of the components of a comprehensive communication assessment is critical to determining the needs that a young child has for early intervention. It is imperative for the early interventionist to determine the communication difficulties that a young child may be having because communication (and language) are an important part of the child's ability to develop relationships with others, to learn about the world, and to become increasingly independent. Table 3-1 provides an overview of the components that will be discussed as part of a comprehensive communication assessment.

INTENTIONALITY

A highlight of a child's becoming a communicator is when the child expresses intentionality. Bates (1979) defined intentional communication as "signaling behavior in which the sender is aware a priori of the effect that a signal will have on his listener and he persists in that behavior until the effect is obtained or failure is clearly indicated" (p. 36).

Wetherby and Prizant (1989) discussed the importance of evaluating both the vertical and horizontal dimensions when assessing if a child's signals are intentional. The vertical dimension reflects the child's progression in the expression of intentionality from being unintentional to the presence of intentionality. Children do not develop intentionality overnight; it is a gradual process that shifts from the use of gestures and vocalizations to the signal intent to the use of language (words). Even before infants can signal

Table 3-1	*Components of a comprehensive communicative assessment*
COMPONENT	**DESCRIPTION**
Intentionality	Criteria to determine intentionality (if a communicative act is intentional): – alternating eye gaze – consistent use or ritualization – persists – modify act Types of communicative intents expressed by young children: – behavioral regulation or requests for objects or actions – joint attention or request for information – declaratives or comments – social interaction

Identification and Analysis of Modes of Expression (Used to Express Communicative Intent)	Types of modes
	1. Vocal
	  – inventory of sounds used
	  – syllable shape
	  – percent of correct consonants
	2. Communicative gestures
	  – conventional
	  – symbolic
	  – nonsymbolic
	  – idiosyncratic
	3. Verbal: Language expression
	  – phonology (intelligibility)
	  – single word utterances
	  – multi-word utterances (analysis of syntax, morphology, semantics, & pragmatic aspects)
	4. Alternative modes of communication
	  – use of signs or sign language
	  – augmentative and alternative communication (specifically object or picture board)
	5. Combination of modes

Caregiver–Infant-Toddler Interaction	Infant-toddler participation – readability or predictability – initiating or responding – turntaking – terminating or topic change Parent (caregiver) participation – responding – synchrony or control
Play	Types of play – schema – functional – symbolic play – parallel or cooperative Relationship between play and language

Continued

Table 3-1 *Components of a comprehensive communicative assessment — cont'd*

COMPONENT	DESCRIPTION
Language Comprehension	Prelinguistic comprehension – response to voice (loud or angry) – response to intonation patterns Linguistic comprehension – response to single words – response to multi-word utterance – response to commands or requests with and without gestures, with and without contextual support
Oral Motor Abilities	Oral motor behavior (including reflex patterns) Feeding
Assessment of Other Sensory Modalities	Hearing Vision

intent, they attempt to share experiences with caregivers by sharing attention and affective states (Stern, 1985) before they develop communicative intentionality and express specific communicative intents. Infants communicate with other individuals without meaning to do so, through the reflexive expression of the infant's internal state. Professionals need to have criteria for deciding when a behavior is considered intentional. Many researchers (Bates, 1979; Harding & Golinkoff, 1979; Scoville, 1983; Wetherby & Prizant, 1989) have contributed to the development of a list of behaviors that would determine if a child's behavior is intentional or not. Included in this list would be the following:

• Alternating eye gaze; coordination of eye gaze between people and desired objects in the environment or the goals the infant wants to accomplish.
• Consistent use or ritualization of the child's own sound or intonation patterns. Ritualization of signals implies conventionalization.
• Persistence in signaling.
• Modification or augmentation of the act if the signal is not having the intended effect on the listener.

The horizontal dimension of intentionality (Wetherby & Prizant, 1989) reflects the infant's ability to communicate for a variety of reasons. Wetherby, Cain, Yonclas, & Walker (1988) indicate that infants and young children use gestures and sounds to communicate for the following reasons:

• To influence another's behavior.
• To attract or maintain another's attention for social interaction.
• To draw joint attention to objects and events.

When assessing communicative intentionality the early interventionist should examine the means through which the infant expresses intent. The means may be a communicative gesture or may consist of other behaviors. Prizant and Wetherby (1993) indicate that "communicative means may include nonverbal and vocal behaviors such as body posture, facial expression, directed gaze and gaze aversion, cry and cooing vocalizations, and intonated vowel and/or babbling vocalizations" (pp. 26-27). Thal and Tobias (1992) also elaborate on what can be included as a communicative gesture. They indicate that a gesture is communicative if it is "accompanied by eye contact, vocalization, or some other physical evidence of an attempt to direct the attention of another person" (p. 1283). However, gestures can be further described as conventional, symbolic, or nonsymbolic. Conventional gestures are non–object related such as shrugging, shaking the head in refusal, and waving "bye-bye." Symbolic gestures are object-related gestures and non-symbolic gestures are deictic gestures, including pointing, showing, and ritualized requests (Thal & Tobias, 1992).

HOW TO ASSESS INTENTIONALITY

Communicative intentionality can be assessed through all of the means (parent or caregiver interview, formal assessment, and informal assessment) that are discussed in Chapter 2. The early interventionist can interview the primary caregiver as to what intents the child expresses and what form is used to express those intents. Formal assessment procedures such as the *Communicative and Symbolic Behavior Scales (CSBS)* (Wetherby & Prizant, 1993) can be administered. Alternatively, the early interventionist can rely on specific items from other formalized assessment instruments such as the *Rossetti Infant Toddler Language Scale* (Rossetti, 1990b). Items such as "reaches upward as a request to be picked up" and "vocalizes a desire for a change in activities" are items from the *Rossetti Infant Toddler Language Scale* that examine this dimension. The early interventionist can observe the child in natural contexts and note the functions expressed and the forms used to express those intents. The early interventionist can also elicit the desired behavior by using elicitation procedures such as the "communicative temptations" (Wetherby & Prizant, 1989) presented in Chapter 2.

PHONOLOGY

There is a relationship between prelinguistic vocal development and words. The relationship between babbling and speech production is controversial because not all agree that the sounds produced prelinguistically are continuous with speech sounds. The discontinuity hypothesis (Jakobsen, 1968) alleges that babbling bears no resemblance to later speech production. In contrast, the continuity hypothesis asserts that babbling gradually shifts from the infant's producing all sounds (universal babbling) to the infant's producing only sounds that are present in the language environment (McLaughlin, 1998). Oller, Levine, Cobo-Lewis, Eilers, and Pearson (1998) indicate that "no person can learn to speak a language effectively without a phonological system and, in particular, without control over canonical syllables" (p. 15). It also appears that the consonants that typically occur in canonical babbling are the same as the early consonants produced in words (Robb & Bleile, 1994; Stoel-Gammon, 1998). These include "predominantly consonant–vowel (CV) syllables that appear to be composed of stop, nasal, and glide consonants (primarily labials and alveolars), and a small number of vowels" (Oller et al., 1998). Proctor (1989) indicates that when examining the characteristics of early phonological development and prelinguistic vocal development and words the interventionist should be aware that there are many sounds in babbling that are not used in real words, that real words may be embedded in babbling, and that some similar sounds and sound structures are found in both. In other words, aspects of both the discontinuity hypothesis and the continuity hypothesis may account for the relationship between early sounds and the phonology of the language. Proctor (1989) indicates that early vocables (phonetically consistent forms) appear to link babbling to meaningful speech.

Infants express intentionality in advance of using words with a combination of vocalizations and gestures. Dromi (1987/1996) indicates that "functionally based pre-linguistic vocalizations are the antecedent behaviors of true words therefore the relationship between these vocalizations and real words must be examined" (p. 14). It is necessary for the early interventionist to be able to accurately describe the phonological system the infant or toddler is using. Masterson and Oller (1999) indicate that, for children who are not yet speaking, interventionists specifically need to examine "the extent to which they (infants) are able to produce well-formed, speech-like vocalizations or babbling" (p. 133). When the child begins to use words a description of the phonology of these words is also needed.

To describe the young child's phonological system (either prelinguistically or linguistically), a sample of the child's speech must be obtained. A variety of methods for obtaining the sample are possible. These include listening to the child live, through an audio or video recording of a speech sample, or through a parent diary or interview. The sample of vocalizations may include both intelligible words and nonconventional vocalizations. Stoel-Gammon (1998) indicates that when children are first acquiring true words, their phonological system has a critical role in the words they will produce. Stoel-Gammon (1998) goes on to say that "the role of phonology declines as vocabulary increases and the influences of the lexicon and phonology become bi-directional" (p. 49). Thus it seems that there are many reasons for the early interventionist to examine a child's phonological system. To examine the vocal development of prelinguistic children, Proctor (1989) indicates that early interventionists should record a sample of the child's vocalizations and then examine the sample in terms of normal stages of vocal development. Proctor (1989) indicates that there are five stages to vocal development. The stages and their highlights as adapted from Proctor (1989) and Proctor and Murnyack (1995) are presented in Table 3-2.

Paul (2001) indicates that typically children with limited expressive vocabularies show small phonetic inventories of consonants and a restricted number of syllable shapes in both meaningful and nonverbal vocalizations. Thal, Oroz, & McCaw (1995) indicate that there are links between a child's lexicon, phonology, and grammar. Specifically, there is a relationship between phonetic inventory and lexicon size (Paul & Jennings, 1992; Thal et al., 1995). Therefore an adequate description of the young child's phonology must be completed as part of a total communication assessment. The description of

| Table 3-2 | *Stages of vocal development: Prelinguistic phonological development* |

STAGE	HIGHLIGHTS
Stage 1: Birth to 1 month— Reflexive	– more crying and discomfort sounds than noncry sounds – crying is reflexive – noncry sounds are vegetative noises (burps, swallows, coughs, etc.); neutral and mainly vocalic (vowel-like) in nature
Stage 2: 1 to 3 months— Cooing	– marked decrease in crying after 12 weeks – vocalic sounds predominate but consonant-like sounds are introduced – approximate velar consonants—combining of consonantal (C) and vocalic (V) segments (coo or goo) – nasalized back vowels – single syllables initially – responds to model of own sound – glottal consonants heard
Stage 3: 4 to 6 months— Babbling	– increased number of C segments produced— more anterior consonants – more variation of V productions – longer syllable sequences, consistent production of CV syllables – vocal play – variations in pitch and loudness
Stage 4a: 7 to 9 months— Reduplicated Babbling	– early nonreduplicated CV syllables – canonical, repetitive, or reduplicated babbling (i.e., CV or CVC-like structure) or repeated consonants across syllables [nanana]) – practice in non-social situations – mama and dada may appear (But is it a word?)
Stage 4b: 10 months— Vocables	– phonetically consistent forms appear to link babbling to speech – context specific – often with gestures
Stage 5: 9 to 18 months— Jargon or Variegated Babbling	– varied sounds and intonation, variety of CV and CVC combinations with sentence-like intonation – resembles sentences – variegated babbling (advanced form of reduplicated babbling), more varied i.e., successive syllables that differ from one another (madagaba)

Adapted from Proctor, A. (1989). Stages of normal vocal development in infancy: A protocol for assessment. *Topics in Language Disorders, 10*, 26-42; and Proctor, A. & Murnyack, T. (1995). Assessing communication, cognition, and vocalization in the prelinguistic period. *Infants and Young Children, 7* (4), 39-54.

the child's phonological system should include a description of the child's consonant inventory, a description of the variety of syllables expressed, and some measure of intelligibility.

Paul and Jennings (1992), adapting the Olswang, Stoel-Gammon, Coggins, & Carpenter (1987) mean babbling level, describe the syllable structure level (SSL) as a measure of the complexity of the child's syllable production. This measure looks at the complexity of the child's syllables in terms of the different combinations of consonants and vowels. Syllable structure is determined by coding and then averaging the levels of a transcribed vocalization using the three levels described in Box 3-1.

Paul and Jennings (1992) found that the average SSL for a 24-month-old child was 2.2 with most vocalizations being coded at level 2 and some vocalizations at level 3. In contrast, Paul and Jennings (1992) reported that toddlers with small expressive vocabulary had an average SSL of 1.7 and that most of these children's vocalizations were coded at level 1 with some at level 2. This information is similar to that of Stoel-Gammon (1991) who indicated that 24-month-old children most frequently used the syllable structure of CV and that this structure was used by 97% of children. Stoel-Gammon (1991) indicates that 97% of the children also used a syllable structure of CVC. Other syllable structures that were used were CVCV (baby, doggie) by 79% of the children and CVCVC (pocket) by 65% of the children.

The early interventionist also needs to determine the child's consonant inventory. Stoel-Gammon (1991) indicates that the child of 24 months should use the following:

- Nine to ten initial consonants.
- Initial consonants: all three places of articulation (labial, alveolar & velar).
- Initial consonants: manner (stop, nasal, fricative, and glide).
- Five or six different final consonants.
- Final consonants: all three places of articulation.
- Final consonants: manner (nasal, fricative, and liquid).

Stoel-Gammon (1991) and Paul and Jennings (1992) reported that 18- to 24-month-olds used 14 different consonants. However, children with small

---

| **Box 3-1** | *Syllable structure level* |

Level 1: The vocalization is composed of a voiced vowel (/a/), voiced syllabic consonant (/l/) or CV syllable in which the consonant is a glottal stop or glide (/ha/ or /wi/).

Level 2: The vocalization is composed of a VC (/up/) or CVC with a single consonant (/kek/) or a CV syllable that does not fit the criteria for level 1. Voicing differences in CVCs are disregarded (toad would be considered a level 2 vocalization).

Level 3: The vocalization is composed of syllables with two or more consonant types, disregarding voicing differences (/pati/ would be level 3 whereas /dati/ would be level 2).

Adapted from Paul, R., & Jennings, P. (1992). Phonological behavior in toddlers with slow expressive language development. *Journal of Speech and Hearing Research, 35,* 99-107. C, Consonant; V, vowel.

expressive vocabularies produced fewer consonants, with the average being six. Stoel-Gammon (1991) reported that children from 24 to 36 months expanded their phonological repertoire and filled in the gaps. Specifically, these children had many more final consonants (9 or 10 final consonants). Paul and Jennings (1992) found that 24- to 36-month-old children produced 18 different consonants and that children of this age with small expressive vocabularies produced only 10 different consonants.

When describing the phonological systems of young children, the early interventionist needs not only to keep the parameters discussed above in mind but also to look for atypical phonological development. Stoel-Gammon (1991) described the following atypical patterns: vowel errors; deletion of initial consonants; substitution of glottal consonants or /h/ for target sounds; substitution of back for front sounds; and deletion of final consonants.

Percentage of correct consonants (PCC) is another procedure that can provide information about the child's phonological system (Shriberg & Kwiatkowski, 1982). The PCC is obtained by transcription of intelligible words, followed by calculation of the mean percentage of correctly produced consonants relative to the adult form of the word. The following question arises: In a child with a limited expressive vocabulary, how many intelligible words are required before this measure can be used? Girolmetto, Pearce, & Weitzman (1997) have used PCC effectively with as few as five words. Paul and Jennings (1992) used PCC with 10 words. Another measure to consider is overall intelligibility of the child's utterances in the total sample. Overall intelligibility is calculated by dividing the number of intelligible utterances by the total number of utterances (including unintelligible and partially intelligible utterances) and multiplying by 100 (Thal, Oroz, & McCaw, 1995).

HOW TO ASSESS PHONOLOGY

As implied above, the speech–language pathologist needs to obtain a speech (vocalization) sample for analysis. The sample should be representative of the child's abilities (remembering the impact that vocabulary has on phonology, the speech–language pathologist needs to interview caregivers to obtain information regarding the words that the child uses communicatively). The sample should be obtained from free play with familiar toys between the child and the caregiver. Transcription of fully intelligible, partially intelligible, and unintelligible utterances (babble) should be completed. A total of 50 to 100 utterances is ideal for analysis.

The focus of intervention with toddlers is language, but within the focus on language Tyler (1996) indicates that it is reasonable to incorporate goals that target the child's phonological system. Bleile (1995) suggests that when the focus of intervention with toddlers is their phonological systems, the focus should be on expansion of the phonetic inventory and syllable structure, and that stimulable sounds be targeted. How does an interventionist determine stimulable sounds when the child's vocabulary is restricted?

Tyler (1996) designed a procedure to assess a toddler's stimulability based on a script-based task that incorporated words selected from a list of common vocabulary items for toddlers and scripted into routines that involved a toy doll. The child's attention is directed to the toy and to the actions, and thus to the target words. Tyler (1996) suggests that assessment of a toddler's phonological stimulability can provide the early interventionist with information on which decisions can be made about which sounds should be targeted for intervention.

VERBAL FORM

It is typically accepted that children begin to use their first words when they are approximately one year of age. The communication assessment should document the words the child uses meaningfully. The interventionist needs to know what criteria to use to determine if the child is using a word meaningfully. To qualify as a true word, the utterance must meet two criteria: It must be used to refer consistently to the same person, object, or event; and it must bear some phonetic resemblance to the adult word (Darley & Winitz, 1961). Size and range of a child's vocabulary are an index of language abilities. Size of vocabulary refers to the number of meaningful words used, and range of vocabulary refers to both the number of different words and the different word classes that are used meaningfully. Nelson (1973) reports that 50% or more of a toddler's vocabulary may be general and specific nominals (nouns). The rest of the child's vocabulary may consist of action words, modifiers, personal–social words, and functional words. In a comprehensive assessment the early interventionist must determine this information. Size and range of a child's vocabulary can be assessed in a number of ways, including parent interview, parent completion of a standardized form such as the *MacArthur Communicative Development Inventories* (Fenson, Dale, Reznick, Thal, Bates, Hartung, Pethick & Reilly, 1993), and direct observation. When assessing a child aged 0 to 3 years, the early interventionist also must remember that typical children begin to combine words into longer units between 18 and 22 months. As the child begins to combine words into multiword utterances, an examination of the child's comprehension and production of grammatical morphemes (e.g., plurals, past tense, and auxiliary verbs) should be completed. In addition, the child's knowledge and use of phrases (noun or verb phrases), different sentence types (questions, negatives, and so forth), and compound or complex sentences must be completed; in other words, an examination of the child's grammar (syntax and morphology) should be conducted. Mean length of utterance should be computed to determine the child's expressive language stage. See Lund and Duchan (1993) and Miller (1981) for a complete review of how to analyze morphology and syntax.

In addition to the description of the form of the verbal language the child uses, a complete assessment encompasses how the child uses his or her linguistic form. Thus information is needed on the pragmatic aspect of language. Communication also involves the organization of conversational discourse (Roth, 1990). The child must function as both a listener and a speaker. The interventionist needs to know how the child uses the linguistic form in initiating and responding to a communicative act, if the child is able to take turns in a communicative exchange, how the child maintains the interaction, and how the child terminates the interaction or changes the topic of the interaction. Information is also needed about the child's ability to provide the amount and type of information that is needed by the listener, as well as the child's use of nonspecific vocabulary, repetition, informational redundancy, and message and situational appropriateness. Assessment of the pragmatic components of communication can be accomplished through structured observations in naturalistic settings. Specific components can be targeted for the observation (e.g., child initiations of conversation), depending on the individual needs of the child.

An analysis of the child's knowledge and expression of the semantic aspect of language also should be incorporated when the child expresses himself or herself with words. Included in the examination of the child's semantics would be examination of the word meaning expressed and understood by the child. This includes determining the number and types of words the child produces and comprehends as well as the meaning relationships expressed within and between sentences. Semantics includes at least three different kinds of meaning. Included would be the lexical meaning or the meaning of words themselves, abstract relational meaning that expresses the relationship between things, and nonliteral meaning or understanding words that are not related to their usual referent but to some characteristic of the referent (Pan & Berko Gleason, 1997). However, a child younger than 3 years would only be expressing lexical meaning and abstract relational meaning. Thus during the assessment the speech–language pathologist also should examine the child's intended meaning of concrete and abstract words as well as the child's understanding of relationships between entities or events (spatial or temporal terms). When the child begins to use multiword utterances, a semantic analysis may include evaluating the child's sentence meaning, which depends on the relationships among the words both within and between sentences. Relational meaning within sentences can include (1) the child's use of a word to describe the relationship between a previous situation and a current situation such as "all gone" after eating a cookie, as well as (2) the child's use of two object labels in combination to describe the relationship between the two objects in the environment such as "Daddy's ball." Relational meaning between sentences includes the child's use and understanding of linguistic devices such as anaphoric and cataphoric referencing, ellipsis, deixis, and lexical cohesion. Assessment of the semantic component of communication can be accomplished through structured observations in naturalistic settings. Specific components can be targeted for observation (e.g., child's expression of early semantic relations) depending on the particular needs of the child.

ALTERNATIVE MODES OF COMMUNICATION

Alternative modes of communication also must be considered in the assessment. Effective communication is essential to a child's social and cognitive development (Prizant & Wetherby, 1993). If a young child has difficulty with verbal or nonverbal self-expression because of cognitive or physical impairments, assistive technology (an augmentative or alternative communication device) may provide that child with a means of developing communicative abilities, overcome communication barriers, or facilitate a link between the child and the daily life experience (Reinhartsen, Edmondson, & Crais, 1997). In particular, when a child's oral–motor abilities are involved and acquiring speech may be delayed, another avenue of expression should be considered. Perhaps the most frequently used alternative methods with communicatively impaired children are the use of signs or sign language and the implementation of a specific augmentative and alternative communication (AAC) technique, such as an object or picture board. An assessment for the appropriateness of using assistive technology or an AAC system with a young child should encompass more than the child's communicative abilities; specifically, the interventionist must consider the child's overall gross and fine motor skills, imitation skills, understanding of object permanence and means–end, attentional skills, motivation for interaction and communication, and level of play (Reinhartsen et al., 1997). The assistive technology or AAC assessment should be completed by a team that specializes in this type of assessment. It is also important for the early interventionist to realize that an augmentative communication system may be a transitional or temporary mode of communication that depends on the individual needs and developmental abilities of the child. Any assistive technology assessment and intervention also should focus on the child and the child's communication partners in the natural environment (Beukelman & Mirenda, 1998). Families at first may be skeptical of early implementation of an AAC system and may need information about the relationship between speech development and AAC system use. Parents and caregivers need to know that the use of an AAC system does not preclude the development of spoken language and that the AAC system may in fact facilitate oral communication and speech.

The reauthorization of IDEA (P.L. 101-476 and P.L. 99-457) emphasizes the need to examine the use of assistive technology to optimize the child's interaction with the environment. AAC systems are a form of assistive technology that facilitates the child's communicative interactions with his or her environment. The AAC assessment should focus on the child and the child's communication partners within natural environments (Beukelman & Mirenda, 1998).

PLAY

Young children engage in pretend play before they learn to talk (Wieder, 1996). Play is critical to the development of language because it provides a social context for interaction and for language learning. Language and play are related in that they have a common cognitive knowledge base (Wetherby, 1992) and both involve the use of symbols. Symbolism is found in language, drawing, gesturing, and play actions (Casby, 1992). There is accumulating evidence of parallels between cognition and the emergence of preverbal communication and first words (McCune, 1986; McCune-Nicolich, 1981). A number of developmental consistencies can be observed in the normally developing child's play and language (Rossetti, 1990a). There seems to be a relationship between young children's play and advances in language, particularly in symbolic play (McCune-Nicolich & Carroll, 1981). Changes in the complexity of play are accompanied by concurrent changes in the child's language abilities (Rossetti, 1990a; Wetherby, 1992). Symbolic play is make-believe play, or the knowledge that one object can be used to represent another. Pretending and language are both based on the capacity to represent, and advances in the complexity of play behaviors are usually accompanied by changes in language use and function in normally developing children (McCune-Nicolich & Carroll, 1981). The sensorimotor–cognitive skills of imitation, tool use, communicative intent, and functional object use were correlated with the emergence of language (Bates, Benigni, Bretherton, Camaioni, & Volterra, 1979). The capacity for symbol use is evident in both the development of language and the development of play. Language provides a tool for engaging others in play, taking on make-believe roles, changing the identity of objects, substituting for actions, negotiating and cooperating with others, and narrating events during play. Language assessment provides the early interventionist with some information about the child's ability to represent the world; an assessment of play is another way in which information about representational capacity can be obtained. Paul (2001) indicates that a play assessment provides a nonlinguistic comparison against which to gauge a child's linguistic performance. For a young child who is communicatively handicapped, a play assessment provides insight into the child's ability to represent, and in the absence of language provides information about the child's potential to learn language. The establishment of a developmental level of play is a reflection of the child's underlying cognitive knowledge. When completing a play assessment the early interventionist is not trying to determine if the child has the "prerequisite" cognitive skills for language use but rather to obtain a total picture of the child's capacity to use symbols and learn symbolic representation. Wieder (1996) indicates that interactive play provides a good opportunity to observe a child's highest level of symbolic functioning. A play assessment may provide the early interventionist with information about the child's (1) understanding of his or her world through analysis of the child's interactions with objects; (2) knowledge of objects, events, relationships between objects and events, and qualities of objects, as well as their location in time and space, through an examination of the child's use of multiple action schemes; and (3) ability to engage in symbolic play.

There are strong ties between symbolic play and language.

- When a child is beginning to display intentional communicative behaviors but not yet using words (presymbolic), the child also is presymbolic in play. The child's play will show exploratory actions with objects, and the child may begin to use objects realistically.
- As the child's language progresses to the use of first words (symbolic behavior), a parallel shift occurs in the child's play in that the child demonstrates symbolic play. The child pretends with realistic objects by using conventional functions toward himself or herself.
- As the child begins to combine words in his or her language, the child's play reflects this increase in symbolic behavior; in play the child demonstrates the ability to combine action schemes together in sequence and to pretend to use these action schemes toward others.

- As the child's symbolic abilities continue to develop, more changes in both language and play are noted. When the child uses many different actions related to a theme and sequences these actions together or pretends without objects, the child uses more and longer sentences.
- Finally, as the child engages in sociodramatic play, takes on a role of someone else, and elaborates the play themes to include peers, the child uses language that is sequenced and discourse based.

HOW TO DO A PLAY ASSESSMENT AND WHAT TO LOOK FOR

Play can be assessed by providing the child with a variety of toys in a natural context and then coding the level of play (Westby, 1988). Westby (1980, 1988) proposed a symbolic play scale that can be used for two purposes: (1) to determine if a child should be given priority for receiving language remediation and (2) if so, to determine what aspects of language (communicative function, semantic concepts, or syntactic structure) should be taught. Using the 1980 scale, Westby indicates that it is when a child's cognitive level is greater than his or her language level that the speech–language pathologist needs to be most concerned. When this occurs, the child is capable of symbol use but has a specific difficulty learning and using language symbols.

McCune-Nicolich (1981) developed a scale that looks at both play and language. Play and language development reflect the child's emerging ability to manipulate symbols. Wetherby (1992) indicates that a play sample should be obtained and the child's play behaviors analyzed (both symbolic play behaviors and constructive play behaviors) to determine at what level the child's play behaviors fall, based on a developmental sequence. Wetherby (1992) suggests that the speech–language pathologist examine symbolic play to understand the child's ability to use symbols.

Wetherby (1992) suggests that it is also important to examine the child's constructive play behaviors. The child who has specific difficulty in symbolic play because of the social or language demands of such play may have strength in constructive play. The child's abilities in constructive play will provide information about the child's mental representational ability and underlying cognitive knowledge.

In addition to the observational formats previously described, some of the formal assessment instruments used to assess a child's play include the *CSBS* (Wetherby & Prizant, 1993), the *Assessing Linguistic Behaviors (ALB)* tool (Olswang et al., 1987), and the *Rossetti Infant Toddler Language Scale* (Rossetti, 1990b). Wetherby and Prizant (1993) incorporate a play assessment into the *CSBS*. The symbolic play probe looks at the child's action schemas (singular or in sequence). This tool also examines the child's combinatorial play abilities by engaging the child in play with specified sets of toys.

The *ALB* tool looks at two categories of play: practice play (actions on objects) and symbolic play (pretend play). The Play Scale in the *ALB* examines the child's practice play during the first year of the sensorimotor period. The child's actions toward objects are observed. In addition, the Play Scale examines symbolic play, which emerges during the second year of the sensorimotor period, and suggests the use of specified sets of toys to elicit play behavior. The *Rossetti Infant Toddler Language Scale* also has a section in which play is examined.

CAREGIVER–CHILD INTERACTION: CAREGIVER VARIABLES

Sociocommunicative skills involve caregiver–infant interaction and attachment, as well as the child's overall ability to comprehend and process language (Rossetti, 1991). The social interaction that takes place between the infant and the caregiver provides the foundation for the child's intentional use of language (Bates, 1979; Bruner, 1981). A comprehensive language assessment should encompass the fact that communication requires two members of a dyad and that it is important to examine both the caregiver–infant interaction and the infant's readiness to communicate.

An important characteristic of early caregiver–child interactions is that the caregiver reads the prelinguistic child's behavior as having communicative value (Wetherby, 1992). A communication exchange takes place every time two or more individuals interact and the behavior of one evokes, maintains, or modifies the behavior of another person (Dunst & Lowe, 1986). Dunst and Lowe indicate that the "extent to which the infant produces distinctive readable behaviors determines to a large degree the manner in which his/her caregivers are likely to respond to the behaviors as intents to communicate" (p. 11). In addition to the importance of the infant's production of readable signals is the extent to which the caregiver can predict the infant's intent. It is within this interaction between caregiver and infant that the infant develops communication. Thus the caregiver's sensitivity and responsiveness within the infant or toddler–caregiver interaction are appropriate targets for communication assessment (Ogletree & Daniels, 1993). The interactive qualities that have been thought to be significant include joint attention, repetitive structure, mutual enjoyment, and sensitivity and responsiveness to the infant's signals (McCollum & McBride, 1997). An examination of the caregiver's end of the interaction should include the following:

- The caregiver's acceptance of the child's communicative attempts.
- The amount, and types, of directives used by the caregiver.
- The caregiver's use of child-oriented strategies (such as responding contingently, providing appropriate communicative models, maintaining the child's communicative topics, and expanding or elaborating on the child's communicative attempts).

A variety of instruments are available to assess these qualities of parent–child interactions, including the following:

- *Parent Behavior Progression* (Bromwich, Khokha, Fust, Baxter, Burge & Kaas, 1981).
- *Observation of Communicative Interaction* (Klein & Briggs, 1987).
- *Parent–Child Interaction Scale* (Farran, Kasari, & Jay, 1983).
- *Mother–Infant Communication Screening* (Raack, 1989).

Munson and Odom (1996) in their review of 17 different rating scales of parent–infant interaction indicate that the "specific purpose for which the assessment information will be used, as well as other contextual variables (e.g., location of the assessment, availability of videotape equipment, and training of staff)" (p. 20) should guide the early interventionist when choosing a caregiver–child interaction assessment instrument.

In addition to the more formal assessment tools previously described, the caregiver–child interaction can be assessed informally. Paul (2001) provided the interventionist with a list of helpful items to observe, which includes the following:

- Pleasure and positive affect.
- Responsiveness to the child's cues of readiness and unreadiness to interact.
- Acceptance of the baby's overall style and temperament.
- Reciprocity and mutuality: the degree to which the parent and infant seem to be in tune with each other.
- Appropriateness of choice of objects and activities for interaction, as well as the parent's awareness of safety issues and choice of activities and objects that interest and engage the baby.
- Language stimulation and responsiveness: the degree to which the mother talks to the baby appropriately, engages in back-and-forth and "choral" babbling activities.
- Encouragement of joint attention and scaffolding of the baby's participation; the extent to which the mother is effective in directing the baby's attention to objects of mutual interest and the ways she evokes progressively more elaborate responses from the baby (p. 224).
- Behaviors to look for in addition to those already listed include mutual enjoyment, balanced turn taking, joint action games (joint action routines), joint referencing, initiation and maintenance of conversational routines or interactions, and use of physical space.

A word of caution is necessary at this point. When examining the caregiver–child interaction, the early interventionist must never make the caregiver feel responsible for the infant's less than expected communication development. The interaction between the caregiver and the child is dynamic and reciprocal. Behaviors of the infant have an impact on behaviors of the caregiver and vice versa; what the interventionist is observing is an artifact of that reciprocal interaction. Another caution deals with the sensitivity of the early interventionist to culturally diverse families. McCollum and McBride (1997) raise the question of whether the same interaction patterns are significant across cultures. Interaction patterns of families from different cultures are based on that family's or culture's perception of disability (Lynch & Hanson, 1998), as well as on the family's goals and values about socialization (McCollum and McBride, 1997; Reynolds and Ingstad, 1995). The early interventionist should remember that there are wide sociocultural variations in terms of who in the family talks or interacts with the child and that there is no optimal or correct communication style. The desired end is a match between the partner's style and the child's ability to participate in the interaction. McCollum and McBride (1997) also indicate that "the parenting behaviors perceived as maladaptive by the majority may in fact be quite adaptive within the contexts in which particular families spend their daily lives" (p. 515). When interpreting results from any measure of caregiver–infant interaction, it is suggested that the evaluator focus on the positive behaviors of the caregiver and infant, and that cultural variation in inter-action patterns be respected.

CAREGIVER–CHILD INTERACTION: CHILD VARIABLES

As stated in the previous section, sociocommunicative skills involve maternal–infant interaction and attachment, as well as the child's overall ability to comprehend and process language (Rossetti, 1991). A comprehensive language assessment should examine both the caregiver–infant interaction and the infant's readiness to communicate. When one assesses the infant's readiness to communicate, the following aspects should be examined: the child's use of gaze, the attention to social stimuli and development of contingency, joint attention and joint action, and affective sharing.

Gaze is a powerful mode of communication. Infants respond to their caregiver's voice and face as early as 2 weeks of age and fixate their gaze on the caregiver's mouth or eyes (Owens, 2001). Infants have been found to have a preference for looking at eyes and the face (McLaughlin, 1998). Reciprocal interactions that involve gaze and vocalizations are natural outcomes of these early preferences for the eyes and face and are found early in the infant's repertoire.

The development of reciprocal social and communicative interaction may depend on the ability to understand contingency (e.g., the fact that actions of others affect one and that one's own actions affect others) (Klinger & Dawson, 1992). Through contingent, predictable, and repetitive interactions with caregivers, infants develop a sense of control over their environments (Lamb, 1981) and begin to perceive themselves as effective social agents (Schaffer, 1977). Thus it is important to examine the contingency between the caregiver and the child. Likewise, the infant needs to be aware that social stimuli may signal the initiation of a communicative exchange.

Another aspect of early communication that should be documented is joint attention. Joint attention includes the triadic exchanges involving the caregiver, the infant, and objects. McLean and Snyder-McLean (1999) indicate that when an adult interacts with an infant the adult attempts to secure the infant's attention to himself or herself or to an object in the environment that they both can focus upon. In these exchanges, caregivers and infants coordinate their attention around objects of mutual interest. Joint attention is observed through the use of referential looking by the child between the object and caregiver (Klinger & Dawson, 1992).

Joint action routines and early routinized interaction games such as peek-a-boo are another important aspect of early communication. Joint action routines provide the infant with the opportunity to learn and practice important aspects of communication (Ratner & Bruner, 1978). In these inter-actions the infant learns about turn taking, as well as event initiation and structure, and because there is a close relationship between what is said and what is done the infant can begin to make sense of the language he or she hears. McLean and Snyder-McLean (1999) indicate that it is in these joint action routines that the infant learns the names for hundreds of objects and events in the child's environment.

Affective sharing involves the interpersonal coordination of affective expression between an infant and his or her caregiver. Typically, the infant and caregiver experience mutual interest and pleasure in each other's smiling and vocalizations (Klinger & Dawson, 1992).

Specifically, the early interventionist should document the child's early interaction skill. Included in this observational documentation should be a description of the following:

- Does the infant engage in reciprocal interactions?
- Does the child attend to another person?
- Does the child attend to or maintain a joint focus of interaction (contextually established, linguistically established)?
- Does the child establish a joint focus or direct another's attention to a focus (entity or event)?
- Does the child fill in a turn (vocally, linguistically, nonlinguistically), and when does the child use multiword utterances to communicate?
- Does the child specify referents not introduced previously?
- Does the child take into account the listener's background knowledge or experience?

LANGUAGE COMPREHENSION

Comprehension is the ability to associate a symbol or sequence of symbols with meaning. Language comprehension must be included in a comprehensive assessment. Thus it is important to assess a child's ability to understand words and word combinations when completing a language comprehension assessment. Comprehension of single words (receptive vocabulary) is correlated with later word production (Bates et al., 1979; Bates, Bretherton, & Snyder, 1988). James (1989) indicates that when assessing language comprehension there are two basic types of comprehension. The first type of comprehension is linguistic comprehension, or the ability to interpret a verbal stimulus using only linguistic cues and linguistic knowledge. The second type of comprehension is communicative comprehension and refers to the ability to interpret a verbal stimuli using all of the information available in the communicative situation. When assessing a child's language comprehension, either linguistic or communicative, the early interventionist should keep in mind that young children often appear to understand words and sentences that are beyond their developmental level. Children may rely on comprehension strategies (Chapman, 1978) to facilitate their comprehension of the total event. Paul (1987) indicates that the comprehension strategies children use to facilitate their understanding change with development, incorporating new linguistic knowledge as it is acquired and integrated with the knowledge of the way things usually happen. The use of comprehension strategies makes the child look good receptively while providing him with a way to interact and with feedback on his performance (Paul, 2001).

When assessing the young child, the early interventionist must remember that language develops within familiar contexts; therefore it is important to note the child's participation in routinized exchanges (interactions) with the caregiver. The child needs to know about the world before he or she can learn language. McLean and Snyder-McLean (1999) present three strategies that infants employ to facilitate their understanding of the world and to help them make sense out of their surroundings. The first strategy used by infants is to "attend to and act on the people and objects in the environment" (p. 82). Thus babies who are in an alert state attend to their environment. The baby watches, listens, touches, and manipulates the people and objects in their environment. This strategy ties into the child's early play skills where the infant is grasping, throwing, tasting, and examining the surrounding objects. The second strategy presented by McLean and Snyder-McLean (1999) is to "observe, listen and learn from other people" (p. 84). It is through the observation of those in their environment that the child seeks to make connections between the world and the language used to mediate that world. In learning from others in the environment the child often uses imitation. Through the reproduction of the actions of others the child modifies his or her own actions. The third strategy presented by McLean and Snyder-McLean is that the child needs to "explore and experiment" (p. 86). The child not only observes, watches, listens, and manipulates objects during interactions with others; the infant is active and seeks out new experiences and knowledge about the world. The infant learns by doing, acting on, and testing out things in the environment.

When assessing the young child between 8 and 12 months of age it is necessary to determine if the child understands a few single words in routinized contexts. It is also important to assess the child's communicative comprehension. To assess communicative comprehension it is necessary to examine the child's understanding of single words paired with nonverbal cues, such as gesturing. At this stage of development the child may use the following comprehension strategies: looking at objects that mother (adult) looks at, acting on objects you have noticed, and imitating ongoing actions.

Between 12 and 18 months of age, the child begins to comprehend single words. Assessment of the child's comprehension of common action words and labels are appropriate targets for assessment at this point (Ogletree & Daniels, 1993). Paul (2001) indicates that when assessing single-word comprehension (linguistic comprehension) the early interventionist wants to determine if the child can comprehend single words without the support of the nonlinguistic context (e.g., without gestures, without eye gaze toward the object, and not supported by the context [in the middle of eating asking for the cup]). The 12- to 18-month-old child also uses comprehension strategies to facilitate his or her understanding. The strategies used by the child include attending to objects mentioned, giving evidence of notice (look or act on what the mother regards), and doing what you usually do (conventional manner) (Chapman, 1978).

The 18- to 24-month old child understands two-word combinations and may understand the words for absent objects (linguistic comprehension). The child still uses comprehension strategies to facilitate his or her communicative comprehension. The strategies the child may use are to locate objects mentioned and give evidence of notice, to put objects in containers or on surfaces, and to act on the object in the way mentioned (the child is the agent). Paul (1987) indicates that in assessing multiword comprehension the early interventionist is interested in determining comprehension of early semantic relations such as agent–object, possessor–possession, action–affected object, and entity–attribute.

Paul (2001) indicates that since the toddler has a comprehension strategy of "do what you usually do," the early interventionist must present two-word instructions that are unexpected and not predicted by context such as "push the apple" when assessing the semantic relation of action–object.

The child between 24 and 36 months of age is able to comprehend three-term sentences, but context and past experience will still have a role. The child does not understand that word order makes a difference in meaning. The comprehension strategies that the child uses include responding with probable locations and using probable events, and supplying the missing information (Chapman, 1978). Paul (2001) indicates that children who succeed at the 24- to 36-month level in a nonstandardized assessment approach that incorporates the information previously described can be assessed using more formalized measures. Formal instruments that assess language comprehension include the following:

- *Peabody Picture Vocabulary Test III* (Dunn & Dunn, 1997).
- *Test of Auditory Comprehension of Language 3* (Carrow-Woolfolk, 1998).
- *Receptive One Word Picture Vocabulary Test* (Brownell, 2000).

Language comprehension is also found in other language assessment instruments that are based on a developmental model of language acquisition. These include the following:

- *Preschool Language Scale 3* (Zimmerman, Steiner & Pond, 2002).
- *Infant Toddler Language Scale* (Rossetti 1990b).
- *Receptive-Expressive Emergent Language Scale III* (Bzoch, League & Brown, 2003).
- *Sequenced Inventory of Communicative Development–Revised* (Hedrick, Prather, & Tobin, 1984)

Comprehension has been found to be a prognostic factor in assessment. Children with better comprehension have better expressive language outcomes (Thal, 1991). Olswang, Rodriguez, & Timler (1998) indicate that the larger the gap between comprehension and production, the poorer the prognosis for language. Thus comprehension is an important aspect of communicative assessment.

ORAL MOTOR ABILITIES

A description of the child's oral motor abilities should include his or her physical ability to produce various sounds, oral motor behavior (including reflex patterns), and feeding patterns. The oral-peripheral examination helps to determine the infant's neurological potential for efficient respiration and feeding and for appropriate, volitional sound production (McCune, Kalmanson, Fleck, Glazewski, & Sillari, 1990). A description of oral motor abilities is crucial to the communicative assessment because the interventionist needs to know if the child's speech development is related to problems in motor speech. A feeding assessment can be used to examine the feeding abilities of an infant as well as to provide information about muscular control and dysarthria-like conditions that could affect speech motor abilities.

It is through a feeding assessment that the speech–language pathologist can obtain information about oral motor behaviors, since it may be difficult to complete a traditional oral motor assessment on a child who is too young to follow commands such as "stick out your tongue" or to imitate. The feeding assessment provides a naturalistic environment to observe structure, function, and tone of the oral motor system. It is also possible during the feeding assessment to note the presence or absence of oral reflexes. The feeding assessment should include the following:

- Comprehensive history of feeding: frequency, amount (see Arvedson & Brody, 2002a, for an example).
- Observation of the child at rest and play (including positioning of the child).
- Tone and reflexes.
- Oral motor exam: presence or absence of oral reflexes; facial expression; symmetry, strength and coordination of lips, tongue, palate, and jaw; control of oral secretions; feeding behavior (including a description of breast or bottle feeding, or both, and types of bottle and nipple used); response to digital stimulation; dental development; breathing, and voice.
- Posture during feeding.

The speech–language pathologist should remember that there are anatomical differences between the oral structures of an infant and an adult. These include the following:

- Jaw (mandible) is small and retracted.
- Space is small.
- Tongue fills oral cavity (tongue is large in relation to cavity).
- Not much oral space is visible.
- Sucking pads add to firmness of cheeks.
- Tongue movement is backward and forward.
- Infants are nose breathers (because there is not enough space in the mouth for air to go in and out).
- Epiglottis and soft palate are in direct approximation.
- Food passes laterally on outside of epiglottis and into esophagus (larynx protects airway and respiration need not be inhibited for swallowing to occur).
- Infants breathe and swallow simultaneously.
- Larynx rides high in neck.
- Eustachian tube is horizontal from middle ear into nasopharynx (Morris & Dunn-Klein, 1987).

Assessment tests of oral motor and feeding issues are commercially available. These include the following:

- *Neonatal Oral-Motor Feeding Scale (NOMAS)* (Braun & Palmer, 1986).
- *Revised version of the NOMAS* (Case-Smith, Cooper, & Scala, 1989).
- *The Pre-speech Assessment Scale* (Morris, 1982).
- *SOMA: Schedule for Oral Motor Assessment* (Reilly, Skuse, & Wolke, 2000).

Evaluation of feeding and swallowing may require the use of additional instrumental procedures such as videofluoroscopic swallow study, flexible endoscopic evaluation of swallowing, and ultrasonographic examination of the oral and pharyngeal cavities. These procedures assist in visualizing the swallowing mechanism in all four phases of the swallow. See Arvedson and Brody (2002b) for a complete description of these procedures.

AUDIOLOGICAL EVALUATION

An audiological screening should also be completed to obtain an estimate of the child's hearing ability and to identify children who should be referred for a complete audiological evaluation. Screening of hearing is an important part of the assessment of all children with suspected speech or language problems. Hearing loss in children can result in speech and language delay, difficulties in parent–child and peer–child interactions, poor academic achievement, and low self-esteem (Carney & Moeller, 1998). Children with developmental delays are at greater risk for hearing loss than children who are developing typically.

Components of hearing screening include a hearing history (history of otitis media) and the infant's reaction to sound. An audiological assessment may include the following:

- Acoustic admittance
- Tympanometry and acoustic reflexes
- Evoked otoacoustic emissions
- Auditory brainstem response (or brainstem auditory evoked response)
- Behavioral audiometry: observation of general awareness of sound, visual reinforcement of audiometry, and conditioned play audiometry

Most of the procedures described above are in the purview of the audiologist. The speech–language pathologist should review the Scope of Practice in Speech–Language Pathology (American Speech–Language–Hearing Association, 2001) for a review of the types of procedures that are appropriate for a speech–language pathologist to administer.

SUMMARY

The components of a comprehensive communicative assessment have been presented in this chapter. See the Appendix for a description of some assessment tools that were referenced in this chapter. In the next chapter, case history information will be presented along with a rationale for an assessment plan and the results of the assessment.

REFERENCES

American Speech–Language Hearing Association (2001). *Scope of practice in speech–language pathology*. Rockville, MD.

Arvedson, J., & Brody, L. (2002a). Clinical feeding and swallowing assessment. In J. Arvedson & L. Brody (Eds.), *Pediatric swallowing and feeding: Assessment and management* (2nd Ed.) (pp. 283-340). San Diego: Singular Publishing Group.

Arvedson, J., & Brody, L. (2002b). Instrumental evaluation of swallowing. In J. Arvedson & L. Brody. (Eds.), *Pediatric swallowing and feeding: Assessment and management* (2nd Ed.) (pp. 341-388). San Diego: Singular Publishing Group.

Bates, E. (1979). Intentions, conventions and symbols. In E. Bates (Ed.), *The emergence of symbols: Cognition and communication in infancy* (pp. 33-68). New York: Academic Press.

Bates, E., Benigni, L., Bretherton, I., Camaioni, L., & Volterra, V. (1979). Cognition and communication from nine to thirteen months: Correlational findings. In E. Bates (Ed.), *The emergence of symbols: Cognition and communication in infancy* (pp. 69-140). New York: Academic Press.

Bates, E., Bretherton, I., & Snyder, L. (1988). *From first words to grammar: Individual differences and dissociable mechanism.* New York: Cambridge University Press.

Beukelman, D., & Mirenda, P. (1998). *Augmentative and alternative communication: Management of severe communication disorders in children and adults* (2nd Ed.). Baltimore: Paul H. Brookes Publishing Co.

Bleile, K. M. (1995). *Manual of articulation and phonological disorders.* San Diego: Singular Publishing Group.

Braun, M. A., & Palmer, M.M. (1986). A pilot study of oral sensorimotor dysfunction in "at-risk" infants. *Physical and Occupational Therapy in Pediatrics, 5,* 13-25.

Bromwich, R., Khokha, E., Fust, L.S., Baxter, E., Burge, D., & Kaas, E. W. (1981). Parent behavior progression. In R. Bromwich (Ed.), *Working with parents and infants: An interactional approach* (pp.341-359). Baltimore: University Park Press.

Brownell, R. (Ed.). (2000). *Receptive one word picture vocabulary test (2000 Edition).* Novato, CA: Academic Therapy.

Bruner, J. (1981). The social context of language acquisition. *Language and Communication, 2,* 155-178.

Bzoch, K. R., League, R., & Brown, V. (2003). *Receptive expressive emergent language scale* (3rd Ed.). Dallas, TX: ProEd.

Carney, A. E., & Moeller, M. P. (1998). Treatment efficacy: Hearing loss in children. *Journal of Speech, Language, and Hearing Research, 41* (Supplement), S61-S84.

Carrow-Woolfolk, E. (1998). *Test of auditory comprehension of language–3.* Dallas, TX: ProEd.

Casby, M. (1992). Symbolic play: Development and assessment considerations. *Infants and Young Children, 4*(3), 43-48.

Case-Smith, J., Cooper, P., & Scala, V. (1989). Feeding efficiency of pre-mature neonates. *American Journal of Occupational Therapy, 43,* 245-250.

Chapman, R. (1978). Comprehension strategies in children. In J. F. Kavanaugh & W. Strange (Eds.), *Speech and language in the laboratory, school, and clinic* (pp.308-347). Cambridge, MA: MIT Press.

Darley, F., & Winitz, H. (1961). Age of the first word: Review of the research. *Journal of Speech and Hearing Disorders, 26,* 271-290.

Dromi, E. (1996). *Early lexical development.* San Diego: Singular Publishing group. (First published in 1987, Cambridge University Press).

Dunn, L. & Dunn, L. (1997). *The Peabody Picture Vocabulary Test–III.* Circle Pines, MN: American Guidance Service.

Dunst, C. J., & Lowe, L. W. (1986). From reflex to symbol: Describing, explaining, and fostering communicative competence. *Augmentative and Alternative Communication, 2*(1), 11-18.

Farran, D., Kasari, C., & Jay, S. (1983) *Parent–Child Interaction Scale.* Chapel Hill, NC: Frank Porter Graham Child Development Center, University of North Carolina.

Fenson, L., Dale, P. S., Reznick, J. S., Thal, D., Bates, E., Hartung, J. P., Pethick, S. & Reilly, J. (1993). *The MacArthur communicative development inventories: User's guide and technical manual.* San Diego: Singular Publishing Group.

Girolmetto, L., Pearce, P., & Weitzman, E. (1997). Effects of lexical intervention on the phonology of late talkers. *Journal of Speech, Language, and Hearing Research, 40,* 338-348.

Harding, C., & Golinkoff, R. (1979). The origins of intentional vocalizations in prelinguistic infants. *Child Development, 50,* 33-40.

Hedrick, D. L., Prather, E., M., & Tobin, A. R. (1984). *Sequenced inventory of communication development* (Revised Ed.). Los Angeles, CA: Western Psychological Services.

Jakobson, R. (1968). *Child language, aphasia, and phonological universals.* The Hague: Mouton. (Original copyright, 1941.)

James, S. (1989). Assessing children with language disorders. In D. K. Bernstein & E. Tiegerman (Eds.), *Language and communication disorders in children* (2nd Ed.) (pp.157-207). Columbus, OH: Merrill Publishing Co.

Klein, M., & Briggs, M. (1987). Facilitating mother–infant communicative interactions in high-risk infants. *Journal of Childhood Communication Disorders, 10* (2), 95-106.

Klinger, L. G., & Dawson, G. (1992). Facilitating early social and communicative development in children with autism. In S. F. Warren & J. Reichle (Eds.), *Causes and effects in communication and language intervention.* Baltimore: Paul H. Brookes Publishing Co.

Lamb, M. (1981). The development of social expectations in the first year of life. In M. Lamb & L. Sherrod (Eds.), *Infant social cognition: Empirical and theoretical considerations* (pp. 155-176). Hillsdale, NJ: Lawrence Erlbaum Associates.

Lund, N., & Duchan, J. (1993). *Assessing children's language in naturalistic contexts* (3rd Ed.). Englewood Cliffs, NJ: Prentice Hall.

Lynch, E. W., & Hanson, J. (1998). *Developing cross-cultural competence: A guide for working with children and their families* (2nd Ed.). Baltimore: Paul H. Brookes Publishing Co.

Masterson, J., & Oller, D. K. (1999). Use of technology in phonological assessment: Evaluation of early meaningful speech and prelinguistic vocalizations. *Seminars in Speech and Language, 20*(2), 133-147.

McCollum, J. A., & McBride, S. L. (1997). Ratings of parent–infant interaction: Raising questions of cultural validity. *Topics in Early Childhood Special Education, 17*(4), 494-519.

McCune, L. (1986). Play-language relationships: Implications for a theory of symbol development. In A. Gottfried & C. C. Brown (Eds.), *Play interactions.* Lexington, MA: Lexington Books.

McCune, L., Kalmanson, B., Fleck, M. B., Glazewski, B., & Sillari, J. (1990). An interdisciplinary model of infant assessment. In S. J. Meisels & J. P. Shonkoff (Eds.), *Handbook of early childhood intervention* (pp. 219-245). New York: Cambridge University Press.

McCune-Nicolich, L. (1981). Toward symbolic functioning: Structure of early pretend games and potential parallels with language. *Child Development, 52,* 785-797.

McCune-Nicolich, L., & Carroll, S. (1981). Development of symbolic play: Implications for the language specialist. *Topics in Language Disorders, 2,* 1-15.

McLaughlin, S. (1998). *Introduction to language development.* San Diego: Singular Publishing Group.

McLean, J., & Snyder-McLean, L. (1999). *How children learn language.* San Diego: Singular Publishing Group.

Miller, J. (1981). *Assessing language production in children.* Boston: Allyn & Bacon.

Morris, S. (1982). *Pre-speech assessment scale.* Clinton, NJ: Preston Publishers.

Morris, S., & Dunn-Klein, M. (1987*). Prefeeding skills: A comprehensive guide to feeding.* Tucson, AZ: Therapy Skills Builders.

Munson, L. J., & Odom, S. L. (1996). Review of rating scales that measure parent–infant interaction. *Topics in Early Childhood Special Education, 16*(1), 1-25.

Nelson, K. (1973). Structure and strategy in learning to talk. *Monographs of the Society for Research on Child Development, 38* (Serial No. 149).

Ogletree, B., & Daniels, D. (1993). Communication-based assessment and intervention for prelinguistic infants and toddlers: Strategies and issues. *Infants and Young Children, 5*(3), 22-30.

Oller, D. K., Levine, S., Cobo-Lewis, A., Eiler, R., & Pearson, B. (1998). Vocal precursors to linguistic communication: How babbling is connected to meaningful speech. In

R. Paul (Ed.), *Exploring the speech–language connection* (pp. 1-23). Baltimore: Paul H. Brookes Publishing Co.

Olswang, L. B., Rodriguez, B., & Timler, G. (1998). Recommending intervention for toddlers with specific language learning difficulties: We may not have all the answers, but we know a lot. *American Journal of Speech–Language Pathology, 3*(7), 23-32.

Olswang, L. B., Stoel-Gammon, C., Coggins, T. E., & Carpenter, R. L. (1987). *Assessing linguistic behaviors.* Seattle: University of Washington Press.

Owens, R. E. (2001). *Language development: An introduction* (5th Ed.). Boston: Allyn & Bacon.

Pan, B. A., & Berko Gleason, J. (1997). Semantic development: Learning the meaning of words. In B. A. Pan & J. Berko Gleason (Eds.), *The development of language* (4th Ed.) (pp. 122-158). Boston: Allyn & Bacon.

Paul, R. (1987). A model for the assessment of communication disorders in infants and toddlers. *NSSLHA Journal,* 88-105.

Paul, R. (2001). *Language disorders from infancy through adolescence: Assessment and intervention* (2nd Ed.). St Louis, MO: Mosby.

Paul, R., & Jennings, P. (1992). Phonological behavior in toddlers with slow expressive language development. *Journal of Speech and Hearing Research, 35,* 99-107.

Prizant, B., & Wetherby, A. (1993) Communication and language assessment for young children. *Infants and Young Children, 5*(4), 20-34.

Proctor, A. (1989). Stages of normal noncry vocal development in infancy: A protocol for assessment. *Topics in Language Disorders, 10,* 26-42.

Proctor, A., & Murnyack, T. (1995). Assessing communication, cognition, and vocalization in the prelinguistic period. *Infants and Young Children,* (4), 39-54.

Raack, C.B. (1989). *Mother–infant communication screening (MICS).* Roselle, IL: Community Therapy Services.

Ratner, N., & Bruner, J. (1978). Games, social exchange and the acquisition of language. *Journal of Child Language, 5*(3), 391-402.

Reilly, S., Skuse, D., & Wolke, D. (2000). *SOMA: Schedule for Oral Motor Assessment.* Eastgardens, New South Wales: Whurr.

Reinhartsen, D. B., Edmondson, R., & Crais, E. (1997). Developing assistive technology strategies for infants and toddlers with communication difficulties. *Seminars in Speech Language, 18,* 283-301.

Reynolds, S., & Ingstad, B. (1995). Disability and culture: An overview. In B. Ingstad & S. R. Whyte (Eds.), *Disability and culture* (pp. 3-32). Berkeley: University of California Press.

Robb, M., & Bleile, K. (1994). Consonant inventories of young children from 8 to 25 months. *Clinical Linguistics and Phonetics, 8,* 295-320.

Rossetti, L. (1990a). *Infant–toddler assessment: An interdisciplinary approach.* Boston: College Hill Publication.

Rossetti, L. (1990b). *Infant Toddler Language Scale.* East Moline, IL: Lingua Systems.

Rossetti, L. (1991). Infant–toddler assessment: A clinical perspective. *Infant–Toddler Intervention: The Transdisciplinary Journal, 1*(1), 11-25.

Roth, F. P. (1990). Early language assessment. In E. D. Gibbs & D. M. Teti (Eds.), *Interdisciplinary assessment of infants: A guide for early intervention.* Baltimore: Paul H. Brookes Publishing Co.

Schaffer, R. (1977). *Mothering.* Cambridge, MA: Harvard University Press.

Scoville, R. (1983). Development of the intention to communicate: The eye of the beholder. In L. Feagans, C. Garvey, & R. Golinkoff (Eds.). *The origins and growth of communication.* Norwood, NJ: Ablex.

Shriberg, L. D., & Kwiatkowski, J. (1982). Phonological disorders III: A procedure for assessing severity of involvement. *Journal of Speech and Hearing Disorders, 47,* 256-270.

Stern, D. (1995). *The interpersonal world of the infant.* New York: Basic Books.

Stoel-Gammon, C. (1991). Normal and disordered phonology in two-year-olds. *Topics in Language Disorders, 11,* 21-32.

Stoel-Gammon, C. (1998). Relationship between lexical and phonological development. In R. Paul (Ed.), *Exploring the speech–language connection* (pp. 25-52). Baltimore: Paul H. Brookes Publishing Co.

Thal, D. (1991). Language and cognition in normal and late-talking toddlers. *Topics in Language Disorders, 11,* 33-42.

Thal, D. A., Oroz, M., & McCaw, V. (1995). Phonological and lexical development in normal and late-talking toddlers. *Applied Psycholinguistics, 16,* 407-424.

Thal, D., & Tobias, S. (1992). Communicative gestures in children with delayed onset of oral expressive vocabulary. *Journal of Speech and Hearing Research, 35,* 1281-1289.

Tyler, A. (1996). Assessing stimulability in toddlers. *Journal of Communication Disorders, 29,* 279-297.

Westby, C. (1980). Assessment of cognitive and language abilities through play. *Language, Speech and Hearing Services in the Schools, 3,* 154-168.

Westby, C. (1988). Children's play: Reflections of social competence. *Seminars in Speech and Language, 9,* 1-14.

Wetherby, A. (1992). *Play development in typical children.* Lockport, NY: EDUCOM Associates.

Wetherby, A. M., Cain, D. H., Yonclas, D. G., & Walker, V. G. (1988). Analysis of the intentional communication of normal children from the prelinguistic to the multi-word stage. *Journal of Speech and Hearing Research, 31*(2), 240-252.

Wetherby, A., & Prizant, B. (1993). *Communicative and symbolic behavior scales.* Itasca, IL: Riverside Publishing.

Wetherby, A., & Prizant, B. (1989). The expression of communicative intent: Assessment guidelines. *Seminars in Speech and Language 10*(1), 77-91.

Wieder, S. (1996). Climbing the "symbolic ladder": Assessing young children's symbolic and representational capacities through observation of free play interaction. In S. J. Meisels & E. Fenichel (Eds.), *New visions for the developmental assessment of infants and young children* (pp. 267-288). Washington, DC: Zero to Three.

Zimmerman, I., Steiner, V., & Pond, R. (2002) *Preschool Language Scale–4 (PLS-4).* Austin, TX: Psychological Corporation.

CHAPTER 4

Case Studies to Illustrate Integration of Assessment Components

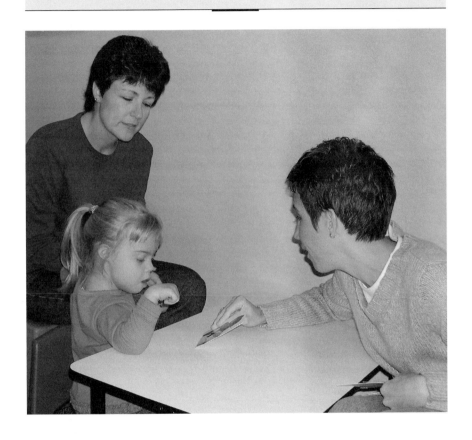

OUTLINE

This chapter presents the reader with case history information concerning children who were referred for early intervention speech and language services. The referral information will be presented and the assessment plan developed; the rationale for the assessment plan will be discussed; and the assessment results, including all information obtained from the interviews, observations, and test administration, will be presented and integrated into a final case summary. This chapter is intended to translate the framework discussed in Chapters 1 through 3 to practical clinical practice.

CASE STUDY 1: JOSHUA P.

J.P. was a 15-month-old boy who was assessed through observation of video-taped interactions made during mother–child play and during an occupational therapy session. J. P. was diagnosed at birth as having Down Syndrome. He was referred for a supplemental speech–language evaluation because of concern about his communication abilities. The following represents a case description provided by the early interventionists who completed the core assessment. The interventionist observed that, in addition to communication problems, J. P. had difficulty on the core battery with visual tracking, fine motor skills, and gross motor skills (a general clumsiness was noted).

J.P. expressed himself through conventional gestures such as requesting, giving, pointing, and limited vocalizations. He comprehended the use of many common objects. He followed simple commands, such as "wash mommy's face," in a routinized face-washing game. He responded to his name and was able to identify objects. When given a choice between a block and a car, he could choose the one named by the adult.

A positive interaction was noted between J.P. and his mother. She commented on his actions and vocalizations in relation to the context. She appropriately labeled objects that J.P. was playing with. However, she employed little use of expansion or extension after labeling objects in the play context.

Assessment Plan

Background Information and Medical History Any past and current medical conditions that might be pertinent to J.P.'s development were investigated. Children born with Down syndrome have an increased incidence of ear infections, respiratory tract infections, and immune deficiency disorders (Tingey, 1988). These conditions would increase J.P.'s risk for hearing and speech problems. In addition, children with Down syndrome may have concurrent cardiac problems or gastrointestinal disorders that may affect normal feeding and swallowing, as well as vocal quality.

Hearing Mild to moderate hearing loss is found in as many as 75% of individuals with Down syndrome (Miller, Leddy, & Leavitt, 1999). Ear infections are a common concern because of enlarged adenoids and tongue, and immune deficiency (Tingey, 1988). Small ear space and hypotonia of the eustachian tube musculature have also been cited (Msall, Digaudio, & Malone, 1991). As a result of these conditions, the hearing of children with Down syndrome tends to fluctuate during early childhood. Due to the high incidence of both conductive and sensorineural hearing loss in children with Down syndrome, a referral for audiological testing should be made.

Vision The referral indicateed that J.P. had visual tracking difficulties. Miller, Leddy, and Leavitt (1999) report that vision problems are common in children with Down syndrome and also indicate that "clinicians need to be sure the children they are testing can see the testing stimuli" (p. 128). Visual tracking and discrimination are important components of social interaction (Ogletree & Daniels, 1993). Thus follow-up in this area is warranted. J.P.'s occupational therapist will be consulted to determine the best methods to monitor J.P.'s visual tracking during the communicative assessment.

Oral Motor Oral anatomical characteristics of some children with Down syndrome include enlarged or protruding tongue, underdeveloped maxilla, narrow palate with broadened alveolar ridges, and enlarged tonsils and adenoids (Tingey, 1988). In addition to these anatomical differences, individuals with Down syndrome are reported to have speech-planning impairments, probably due to underlying nervous system variations that impact oral motor movements (Leddy, 1999). A complete oral motor examination is indicated in these cases.

Play Play is related to language (Westby, 1988; Wetherby, 1992). Fewell, Ogura, Notari-Syverson, and Wheeden (1997) specifically indicate that play and communication are related in young children with Down syndrome. No information was given about J.P.'s play skills. Therefore an assessment of both his symbolic and constructive play skills is warranted.

Communication Assessment of communication abilities should take place in familiar situational contexts over time and should encompass several means for obtaining information (Wetherby & Prizant, 1993). The inclusion of caregivers is also critical, if the assessment is to follow the principles outlined in Chapter 2. Thus J.P. was observed in his most comfortable environment, his home, engaged in play interactions with his mother (his primary caregiver). Mrs. P. has indicated that she was uncomfortable being videotaped; therefore the interventionist compiled observations and administered the *Rossetti Infant Toddler Language Scale* (Rossetti, 1990).

Mundy, Kasari, Sigman, and Ruskin (1995) indicate that measures of nonverbal communication are important in describing the links between nonverbal and verbal communication in children with Down syndrome. Young children with Down syndrome are reported to display strength in the expression of nonverbal social interactive communicative intents and less ability in the expression of behavior regulation (communicative intent used to request) (Mundy et al., 1995; Mundy, Sigman, Kasari, & Yirmiya, 1988; Weitzner-Lin, 1997). To have a complete picture of J.P.'s communicative abilities, a complete description of his nonverbal communicative behaviors as well as his verbal communicative behaviors was needed, with particular emphasis on his expression of a range of communicative functions.

Communication temptations were used to obtain information about how J.P. communicates and why he communicates.

Assessment Results

J.P. is a 15-month-old male who was referred for a supplemental speech–language evaluation. An understanding of J.P.'s communication status was gained through parental report, informal observation, and administration of the *Rossetti Infant Toddler Language Scale.*

Background Information and Medical History J.P. is a 15-month-old male with Down syndrome who lives with his parents, Mr. and Mrs. P., and his 5-year-old sister, Johanna. Mrs. P. reported that J.P. was born full term following an uneventful pregnancy and delivery. At one month, an electrocardiogram and a chest radiograph were obtained to determine J.P.'s cardiac status. Results indicated that J.P. had normal cardiac functioning. No gastrointestinal complications were reported, and Mrs. P. stated that J.P. has no feeding concerns. J.P. has been treated with oral antibiotics for otitis media with effusion. The most recent incident was at 13 months. At this time, J.P. was not taking any medications.

Formal Test Results J.P.'s formal test results on the *Rossetti Infant Toddler Language Scale* are shown in Table 4-1.

Receptively, J.P.'s age equivalent was 9 to 12 months with some scatter skills up to the 12- to 15-month level. J.P. was able to participate in speech routine games, to identify three body parts (hair, nose, and eyes) on himself and to identify eyes and nose on a stuffed animal, and to look at or attend to objects and people when named or mentioned in a conversation, and he appeared to understand simple questions. He responded to a "give me" command and occasionally followed other simple commands. The only item

Table 4-1	*J.P.'s results: Rossetti Infant Toddler Language Scale*	
TEST	BASAL	CEILING
Interaction or attachment	9-12 mo	18-21 mo N/A
Pragmatics	9-12 mo	18-21 mo
Gesture	9-12 mo	15-18 mo N/A
Play	9-12 mo	15-18 mo
Language comprehension	9-12 mo	15-18 mo
Language expression	6-9 mo	15-18 mo

on the 12- to 15-month level that was demonstrated was his shaking his head to say "no." He had not yet evidenced the following skills up through his chronological age level: to point to two action words in pictures, to understand prepositions, and to respond to requests to say words.

An expressive age equivalent of 6 to 9 months was also attained with some emerging skills at the 9- to 12-month level. J.P.'s vocalizations included /duh/, /buh/, /bah/, and /nah/, as well as /uhoh/. He was beginning to imitate some environmental sounds (e.g., motor, animal sounds) during play. In addition, he imitated /lalalala/ as part of a song. He was not observed or reported to imitate or spontaneously produce single words, to intersperse true words within jargon, or use only words as opposed to gestures or gestures and vocalizations to communicate.

J.P. participated in speech routine games, played peek-a-boo, and explored new toys when presented. He waved bye-bye and showed, pointed, and reached to communicate.

Informal Observations J.P.'s play skills appeared appropriate for very familiar toys (he pushed a truck, threw a ball, and turned pages in a book). He was able to stack a two-block tower after modeling. He was not interested in feeding or grooming a doll or stuffed animal.

J.P.'s primary mode of communication was pointing. In addition, he used other gestures such as reaching, smiling, and directed eye gaze. He used limited vocalizations.

The vocalizations were primarily open vowels or consonant–vowel (CV) syllables where the consonant is a /d/, /b/, or /n/. His use of vocalizations was limited. He specifically used vocalizations to direct the adult's attention and to refuse an event or object. J.P. was able to initiate and maintain social interactions during a routinized social object game. He was able to initiate and maintain joint attention through gestures and eye gaze.

J.P. used all his forms of communication to comment on objects in his environment (to name people and objects). He used eye gaze alone or in combination with a vocalization to obtain adult attention. He requested objects by combining pointing and eye gaze. While interacting with his mother, J.P. was able to initiate, maintain, repair, and terminate interactions.

A positive interaction was noted between J.P. and his mother. Mrs. P. commented on J.P.'s actions and vocalizations in relation to the context. She appropriately labeled objects with which J.P. was playing. However, she employed little use of expansion or extension after labeling objects in the play context.

Oral Motor and Feeding An informal oral peripheral examination was performed, and J.P.'s skills were judged to be within normal limits. Low tone of the tongue and cheeks was noted; J.P. was able to control tongue movement, but a slight open mouth posture (no tongue protrusion) was observed at rest. No feeding concerns were reported or observed. He typically ate in a high chair using his fingers, and he drank from a cup (with or without a lid).

Hearing J.P. had not had a formal hearing evaluation. Informal observation indicated that he could localize speech and sound. Mrs. P. reported that J.P. had had several middle ear difficulties. The family was still waiting for an audiological evaluation.

Early-Intervention Evaluation Findings Evaluation findings in the areas of cognitive abilities, adaptive skills (self-help, fine motor, and gross motor), and social and emotional abilities indicated that J.P. was eligible for services because of his diagnosis and that he exhibited mild delays in self-help skills (dressing), gross motor skills (unable to creep upstairs), and fine motor skills (putting pegs in hole).

Summary J.P. presented at least a 3- to 6-month delay in language comprehension and a 3- to 9-month delay in other components of language, with the most significant delay in the area of expressive language. J.P.'s phonological skills were also delayed. Due to J.P.'s diagnosis of Down syndrome, he was eligible for services intended to reduce developmental delays and to lessen additional delays in the future.

At the individualized family service plan (IFSP) meeting, Mrs. P. stated that she wanted J.P. to receive special education services and speech–language services twice a week in the home. She also stated that the outcome she desired would be for J.P. to talk as well as other children his age.

Conclusions

At 15 months of age J.P. expressed a variety of communicative intentions; however, he had limited vocalizations. Paul (2001) reported that children with little speech who do communicate with those around them have a potentially strong foundation that can support functional language growth. In addition, J.P.'s age-appropriate play skills (his constructive play level, stacking a two-block tower, represents an age level of 1 to $1^1/_2$ years) were a good indicator that he has the potential to use spoken words.

CASE STUDY 2: BRANDON Z.

In New York State, it is not unusual for the speech–language pathologist to receive a case like that which follows.

B.Z. was a 26-month-old boy who was assessed through observation of a play session involving him and his mother. He had been referred for a supplemental speech–language evaluation because of concern about his communication abilities. The following represents a case description provided by the early interventionists who completed the core assessment. The interventionist observed that, in addition to communication problems, B.Z. had difficulty on the core battery with visual tracking and fine motor skills; a general clumsiness of gross motor skills was noted.

The core battery reported that B.Z. expressed himself through gestures and vocalizations. In addition, he was able to identify a few body parts by name. B.Z. understood simple commands such as "put away" when embedded in a clean-up routine.

A positive interaction was noted between B.Z. and his mother. Mrs. Z. commented on B.Z.'s actions and vocalizations in relation to the context. She appropriately labeled objects with which B.Z. was playing. However, she employed little use of expansion or extension after labeling objects in the play context.

Assessment Plan

To permit a complete assessment of B.Z.'s communication abilities, the speech–language pathologist must be able to describe in detail the next step in the assessment process for B.Z., obtain the information that is needed, clearly explain why it is needed, and describe how that information will be collected.

A comprehensive speech and language assessment should begin with the obtaining of medical background information. Medical records are potentially an important source of information (Rossetti, 1990; Shipley & McAfee, 1992).

Background Information and Medical History Case history information should also be reviewed. This information can influence the selection of assessment materials.

Communication At 26 months, B.Z. should have been using words and word combinations to communicate; however, it was reported that he communicated only through gestures and vocalizations. Information was needed regarding B.Z.'s communication skills. Wetherby and Prizant (1989) indicated that children with disabilities rely primarily on gestures because they have difficulty expressing their communicative intentions with verbalizations.

Since B.Z. communicated through gestures and vocalizations, it was necessary to investigate the frequency and diversity of the communicative intents B.Z. expressed. Paul (2001) reported that even before children talk, they communicate with those around them. Assessment of expression of communicative intent can be accomplished in two ways: through observation of low-structured interactions in which interesting toys are made available to the child or through the use of communicative temptations (Wetherby & Prizant, 1993). Both methods were used to obtain information about B.Z.'s communicative abilities. Various communication temptations from the *Communication and Symbolic Behavior Scales (CSBS)* (Wetherby & Prizant, 1993) were administered. The communicative temptations provided information about the range of communicative functions expressed, the frequency and diversity of communicative intents expressed, and the form of this communication.

A speech and language sample was also collected, and a complete description of the forms B.Z. used to communicate was completed. Included in this report was a description of B.Z.'s phonological skills. Stoel-Gammon (1998) reported that there is a close relationship between the development of words and sounds in young children. The speech and language sample also included a description of B.Z.'s lexical production because developing children between 18 and 36 months of age usually produce some intelligible words (Paul, 2001). In addition, the speech and language sample was inspected for the use of two-word combinations.

Speech Production A complete analysis of B.Z.'s phonology was needed because there is accumulating evidence that links exist between phonology and grammar (Thal, Oroz, & McCaw, 1995) in late talkers. B.Z. used vocalization during the initial assessment. More information was needed about whether B.Z.'s vocalizations were approximations of words or if his level of speech production was prelinguistic. Analysis included a description of the consonants B.Z. used. Syllable structure level (SSL) (Paul & Jennings, 1992) was used to measure the complexity of B.Z.'s syllable production. B.Z.'s speech motor development also had to be examined.

Language Comprehension The case history indicated that B.Z. was able to identify body parts and to follow simple commands embedded in a familiar routine. Additional information about B.Z.'s comprehension was needed; his receptive language was analyzed to determine if he had an isolated language production deficit or a more pervasive language disorder.

Play The case description did not mention anything about B.Z.'s play skills. Play skills are an important part of the assessment process, as play level may reflect a child's language development (McKimmey, 1993). Paul (2001) indicated that behaviors observed in a child's play tend to go along with communication development. In particular, changes in symbolic play reflect changes in language use. Furthermore, children's symbolic play relates to cognition, socialization, literacy, and language (Westby, 1988). Therefore B.Z.'s play skills were also evaluated through informal observation and parental report.

Oral Motor Oral motor development was also subject to evaluation. B.Z. appeared to have slow speech development, and it was helpful to determine whether this condition was related to a deficit or delay in speech motor abilities (Paul, 2001). Oral motor skills were assessed through informal observation of the oral mechanism while B.Z. ate and drank, and through imitation of oral motor movements.

Hearing As part of the speech and language evaluation B.Z. was referred for a complete audiological evaluation.

Other Areas In response to the difficulty reported with visual tracking, fine motor skills, and a general clumsiness of gross motor skills, it was suggested that B.Z. be referred for an occupational therapy evaluation. In addition, a vision screening was warranted.

Assessment Results

B.Z. is a 26-month-old male who was referred for a supplemental speech–language evaluation. An understanding of B.Z.'s communication status was gained though parental report, informal language sampling (including administration of various communication temptations from the *CSBS*), and observation, as well as administration of the *Receptive-Expressive Emergent Language Scale II* (Bzoch & League, 1991). B.Z.'s background information and medical history were the same as those reported on the core assessment.

Formal Test Results B.Z.'s receptive age equivalent was determined to be 14 to 16 months with some scatter skills up to 24 months. B.Z. was able to identify four body parts by name (hair, nose, eyes, and mouth), associate words by categories (understood that horse and cow are animals, and that fork and spoon are silverware), and demonstrate understanding of action words ("throw," "kiss," and "sit"). He had not demonstrated the following skills up through his chronological age level: to follow two- and three-step consecutive related directions, understand distinctions in personal pronouns, and understand more complex language (including word associations).

An expressive age equivalent of 14 to 16 months was also attained, with some emerging skills at the 18- to 20-month level. B.Z. was reported to produce 7 to 10 words or word approximations and produced only the consonants /t/, /d/, and /n/. He was beginning to imitate some environmental sounds (i.e., motor, animals) during play. He was not observed or reported to imitate or spontaneously produce successive single words or two- or three-word utterances, to intersperse true words within jargon, or to use only words as opposed to gestures or gestures and words to communicate.

Informal Observations A speech and language sample was collected during play interactions with both the speech–language pathologist and B.Z.'s mother. In addition, communication temptations were completed.

B.Z.'s primary mode of communication was pointing. In addition, he used other gestures such as reaching, smiling, and directed eye gaze. He used limited vocalizations. Many vocalizations consisted primarily of open vowels. Word approximations were noted and they were either CV or VC with an occasional CVC and CVCV* syllable shapes. A more complete description of B.Z.'s speech during communicative temptations and a few play interactions is given in Table 4-2.

Analysis of B.Z.'s verbalizations indicated that his SSL was 2 (Paul & Jennings, 1992). The total number of different consonants was seven, with five consonants used in the initial position and three different consonants used in the final position.

Analysis of the informal language sample and the communication temptations indicated that B.Z. used word approximations to comment on objects

---

*CV, Consonant-vowel; VC, vowel-consonant; CVC, consonant-vowel-consonant; CVCV, consonant-vowel-consonant-vowel.

Table 4-2 *B.Z.'s speech during communicative temptations and play interactions*

VERBALIZATION	SSL	INITIAL CONSONANT	FINAL CONSONANT	ADULT GLOSS
/don/	3	/d/	/n/	"down"
/ʌh dis/	3	/d/	/s/	
/dʌdʌ/	2	/d/		maybe "daddy"
/aet/	2		/t/	maybe "cat"
/oudit/	2		/t/	
/whʌdit/	3	/wh/, /d/	/t/	maybe "what this"
/dʌ/	1	/d/		
/da/	2	/d/		
/hʌ/	1	/h/		
/bʌ/	2	/b/		maybe "Brandon"
/nae/	2	/n/		maybe "mom"

in his environment (to name people or objects). He used eye gaze alone or in combination with a word approximation to obtain adult attention ("da" to call dad). B.Z. requested objects by combining pointing and eye gaze. While interacting with his mother, B.Z. was able to initiate, maintain, repair, and terminate interactions.

B.Z. used fewer than 10 words or word approximations during the evaluation. Mrs. Z. reported that the number and types of words used during the evaluation were commensurate with his productions at home.

B.Z.'s play skills were judged to be age appropriate as well as supportive of word combinations (Westby, 1988; Wetherby, 1992). During play interactions B.Z. combined two related sequences (stirred food and then fed the baby with a spoon). He also demonstrated a longer play episode when he picked up the toy phone, vocalized, and then handed the phone to his mother. B.Z. also played appropriately with several other toys (e.g., pushed a toy car, threw a ball).

An informal oral examination was performed and B.Z.'s skills were judged to be within normal limits. B.Z. ate a snack of cheese and crackers and drank apple juice from a cup with adequate lip closure. Mrs. Z. reported that B.Z. typically sat in a booster seat and used a spoon or his fingers to eat. He drank from a cup both with and without a lid without spilling.

A hearing screening was attempted but B.Z. was reluctant to participate. Mrs. Z. reported that there had been no middle ear difficulties, but a referral to an audiologist for a complete hearing assessment was warranted.

Results of the occupational therapy evaluation and the vision screening were not available.

Summary B.Z. presented at least a 10- to 12-month delay in both expressive and receptive language skills. B.Z.'s phonological skills were significantly delayed. B.Z. was eligible to receive speech and language early intervention services.

Conclusions

At 26 months, the shapes of B.Z.'s syllables were slightly below age level. Paul (2001) reported that typically developing 24-month-olds have an SSL of 2.2 with most utterances at level 2 and some at level 3. B.Z.'s overall SSL was slightly below the 24-month level, but he did show a range of syllable types. B.Z. only produced five different initial consonants and three different final consonants. According to Stoel-Gammon (1991), typically developing children produce 9 or 10 different initial consonants and 4 or 6 different final consonants. Thus it can be said that B.Z.'s consonant inventory was significantly reduced.

B.Z. expressed a variety of communicative intentions. Paul (2001) reported that children with little speech who do communicate with those around them have a potentially strong foundation that can support functional language growth. In addition to B.Z.'s strong play skills, the prognosis for functional language development was good.

REFERENCES

Bzoch, K. R., & League, R. (1991). *Receptive-Expressive Emergent Language Scale* (2nd Ed.). Dallas, TX: ProEd.

Fewell, R. R., Ogura, T., Notari-Syverson, A., & Wheeden, C. A. (1997). The relationship between play and communication skills in young children with Down syndrome. *Topics in Early Childhood Education, 17*(1), 103-118.

Leddy, M. (1999). Biological bases of speech. In J. F. Miller, M. Leddy, & L. A. Leavitt (Eds.), *Improving the communication of people with Down syndrome* (pp. 61-80). Baltimore: Brookes.

McKimmey, M. A. (1993). Child's play is serious business. *Children Today, 22*(2), 14-15.

Miller, J. F., Leddy, M., & Leavitt, L. A. (1999). *Improving the communication of people with Down syndrome*. Baltimore: Brookes.

Msall, M. E., DiGaudio, K. M., & Malone, A. F. (1991). Health, developmental, and psychosocial aspects of Down Syndrome. *Infants and Young Children, 6*, 35-45.

Mundy, P., Kasari, C., Sigman, M., & Ruskin, E. (1995). Nonverbal communication and early language acquisition in children with Down syndrome and in normally developing children. *Journal of Speech and Hearing Research, 38*(1), 157-167.

Mundy, P., Sigman, M., Kasari, C., & Yirmiya, N. (1988). Nonverbal communication skills in Down syndrome children. *Child Development, 59*, 235-249.

Ogletree, B. T., & Daniels, D. B. (1993). Communication-based assessment and intervention for prelinguistic infants and toddlers: Strategies and issues. *Infants and Young Children, 5*(3), 22-30.

Paul, R. (2001). *Language disorders from infancy through adolescence: Assessment and Intervention* (2nd Ed.). St Louis, MO: Mosby.

Paul, R., & Jennings, P. (1992). Phonological behavior in toddlers with slow expressive language development. *Journal of Speech and Hearing Research, 35*, 99-107.

Rossetti, L. (1990). *Infant Toddler Language Scale*. East Moline, IL: Lingua Systems.

Shipley, K. G., & McAfee, J. G. (1992). *Assessment in speech–language pathology: A resource manual*. San Diego: Singular.

Stoel-Gammon, C. (1991). Normal and disordered phonology in two-year-olds. *Topics in Language Disorders, 11*, 21-32.

Stoel-Gammon, C. (1998). Relationship between lexical and phonological development. In R. Paul (Ed.). *Exploring the speech–language connection* (pp. 25-52). Baltimore: Brookes.

Thal, D., Oroz, M., & McCaw, V. (1995). Phonological and lexical development in normal and late-talking toddlers. *Applied Psycholinguistics, 16*, 407-424.

Tingey, C. (1988). *Down syndrome: A resource handbook.* Boston: College Hill Press.

Weitzner-Lin, B. (1997). A comparison of intentional communication in children who have Down syndrome with typical children matched for developmental and chronological age. *Infant-Toddler Intervention: The Transdisciplinary Journal, 7*(2), 123-132.

Westby, C. (1988). Children's play: Reflections of social competence. *Seminars in Speech and Language, 9,* 1-14.

Wetherby, A. (1992). *Play development in typical children.* Lockport, NY: Educom.

Wetherby, A., & Prizant, B. (1989). The expression of communicative intent: Assessment guidelines. *Seminars in Speech and Language, 10*(1), 77-91.

Wetherby, A., & Prizant, B. (1993). *Communicative and Symbolic Behavior Scales.* Itasca, IL: Riverside.

CHAPTER 5

General Considerations in Intervention

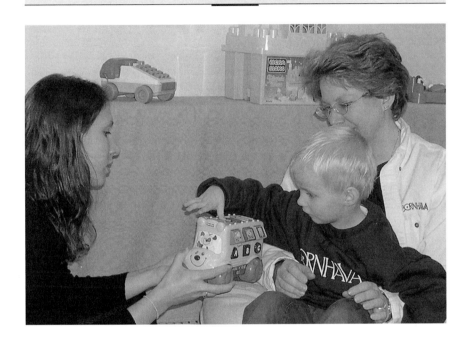

OUTLINE

GENERAL GUIDELINES	INDIVIDUAL FAMILY SERVICE PLANS
INTERVENTION OUTCOMES	GUIDELINES FOR EFFECTIVE HOME VISITS
CONTEXT OF INTERVENTION	BUILDING SUPPORT NETWORKS

This chapter presents a pragmatic/interactionist framework for communication intervention with young children that is based on best practices for early intervention as mandated by federal law.

GENERAL GUIDELINES

Before intervention is begun with infants and toddlers at risk for communication delays, or infants and toddlers who are communicatively impaired, some general guidelines must be developed for providing that intervention. An overall goal for early intervention should be to bolster infants and toddlers in "being and doing-being with people who they want and need to be with and doing what they want and need to do" (Sheldon and Rush, 2001, p. 2). In keeping with the orientation of this text, which is a parent-focused approach to early intervention, the early interventionist should develop early intervention outcomes and goals based on the family's needs and priorities. Being family focused means that families are placed in the center of all services and supports. Intervention outcomes put infants and caregivers in touch with one another while facilitating the infant's competence. The communication outcomes may focus on the child, the caregiver, the interaction, or any combination of these (Sparks, 1989). These outcomes should be derived from the family's needs and priorities, not from the interventionist's assessment. In other words, these goals are family goals or outcomes, not specifically child goals or outcomes. In addition to outcomes that are family focused, the context in which the intervention takes place must be natural and family centered. Lastly, the intervention strategies employed in the natural environment to produce the outcomes and meet the goals should be caregiver friendly.

Another intervention guideline is that the early intervention team must be flexible. "Providing opportunities for parents to talk about changes in their lives and listening carefully to what they say will usually supply professionals with information about changes in family priorities" (McWilliam, 1996a, p. 154). Flexibility is multifaceted; it can stem from the family's priorities, or it can be based on procedural issues such as changes to the time of service provision or transportation issues.

McWilliam (1996a) suggested that the early interventionist should emphasize the positive. Parents or caregivers generally want to do what is best for their child, and giving the family a compliment can do more toward developing a respectful working relationship with the family than any list of suggested things to do when working with families.

INTERVENTION OUTCOMES

The outcomes of intervention that are presented in the individual service plan are parent initiated. These outcomes, as stated earlier, can focus on the infant or toddler, the interaction, or the parent's participation in the process. Whatever the focus, the outcomes should be functional for the child and the family, as well as priority behaviors for the family (Donahue-Kilburg, 1992, p. 243). The specific intervention outcomes must be developmentally appropriate. Thus the targets are chosen for their importance to the interaction between the child and the caregiver. Owens (1999) indicated that the "language development of typical children can guide the selection of intervention targets." However, he also advises the interventionist that strict adherence to a developmental hierarchy may be unsuitable because the interventionist needs to follow the child's individual productive strategies. The interventionist also needs to keep in mind that the communication targeted for the child is not only developmentally appropriate but also fitting for the child's everyday context(s). However, because language is influenced by the context, the targeted communication may be context appropriate but not developmentally appropriate. The child's knowledge of the event, situation, routine, or activity influences the manner in which the child uses language in that context (Owens, 1999). A 2-year-old child does not talk about a recent dinner at grandma's house while playing ball, but may in fact say "hit ball," even though he or she does not use past tense in any other context.

Communicative intervention goals should be based on the child's area of need, and these outcomes may change depending on whether the child is prelinguistic, emerging linguistic, or linguistic. Prelinguistic intervention outcomes may focus on feeding and oral motor development, parent–child interaction, vocal development, and development of communicative intent. Paul (2001) indicates that the communicative intervention goals for the emerging language user should address one or more of the following areas: development of symbolic play skills; use of intentional communicative behavior; language comprehension; and production of sounds, words, and word combinations. Intervention outcomes for the child developing language or for the preschool child may focus on phonology, semantics, syntax and morphology, pragmatics, comprehension, and play and thinking (Paul, 2001). These intervention outcomes should help the child acquire intelligible, grammatical, and flexible forms of expression for the ideas and concepts the child has in mind, as well as give the child tools to make communication effective, efficient, and rewarding so that social interaction proceeds as normally as possible (McLean, 1989; Paul, 2001).

Intervention outcomes and plans should be prioritized so that it is possible to translate the desired outcomes, strategies, and activities into daily practice. Hanson and Bruder (2001) suggested that "embedding children's goals and objectives (outcomes) in routine and play activities should be a generalized approach adopted by all early intervention personnel" (p. 24). These routines and play activities can occur in many different locations, so that when the early intervention team develops family outcomes, the context of the intervention or the locations in which intervention is to occur should be considered. In addition to incorporating family rituals and routines and child play activities, intervention must fit the family's lifestyle. If the intervention strategies fit naturally into the family's participation in the family ritual or routine, and if what is being asked of the family can easily be part of that ritual or routine, the intervention might not be a burden for the family.

CONTEXT OF INTERVENTION

Providing intervention in natural contexts not only is the focus of this text but also is mandated by the 1997 amendments to Part C of the Individuals with Disabilities Education Act (1997). In this law, natural environments are defined as "settings that are natural or normal for the child's age peers who have no disabilities." Many factors influence the decision about the optimal environments in which early intervention will take place. These include "location of the family's home, needs of the child, the resources of the family and the community, and the recommendation of the IFSP team" (Hanson & Bruder, 2001, p. 52). Natural environments or ordinary life situations have been thought to include "play, physical care, and activities of everyday life as parents learn to parent their special-needs child with pleasure and success" (Hershberger, 1991, p. 83). These environments can include a variety of places in addition to the infant's or toddler's home. Dunst, Trivette, Humphries, Raab, and Roper (2001) indicated that the contexts for intervention are not a "deliberate curriculum" but occur in ordinary life situations that are the "who, what, where, when and why of daily life." Natural environments can include playgrounds, fast food restaurants, grocery stores, and even family cars (Bruder and Dunst, 2000). When intervention takes place in these natural environments the interventionist should realize that where service is provided depends on what must be done as well as where the family wants the service to occur.

Thinking about the context of the early intervention is multifaceted. The interventionist needs to take the following factors into consideration:

- Where intervention takes place and the child's functioning in the natural context.
- Family routines.
- Developmental appropriateness of the "where."
- Planned or unplanned events.
- Involvement or participation in the event.
- Manipulation of the event.
- Event structure.

When the early interventionist plans where intervention should take place, several additional factors should be taken into consideration. First, the interventionist needs to know how the child really functions in his or her natural environments, which in turn leads to what the child needs to know in order to function maximally in those environments. How does the interventionist determine real functioning in real environments? The interventionist needs to observe the child within his or her natural environments and to interact with the child's primary caregiver or family members to determine what is important to them. Asking the caregivers to describe their daily routines and, more importantly, the child's participation in those routines and activities should lead to intervention outcomes. Hanft and Pilkington (2000) suggested that the interventionist needs to answer questions such as the following: What dressing and feeding tasks reinforce perceptual and motor competencies? Which household items and toys promote developmental skills? Which playmates, toys, and furnishing encourage a toddler's physical exploration and verbal expression? (p. 4). The answers to questions such as those just presented should reduce the interventionist's dependence on a specific place for intervention and increase the realization that providing intervention in the child's natural environment is the best way to increase that child's play, motor, cognitive, communicative, and social–emotional capabilities.

The interventionist needs next to determine the specific context in specific environments that will facilitate the child's abilities. These specific environments enhance the contextual learning. "Contextual learning can be described as learning that enables a child to participate in activities that are familiar and meaningful, both socially and culturally relevant" (Roper & Dunst, 2003, p. 216). When considering specific contexts within specific environments, the interventionist should ensure that the activity is appropriate to the family (e.g., the context in which the child spends time [the home, daycare]), and is both developmentally and age appropriate for the infant or toddler. In addition, Dunst, Bruder, Trivetee, Hamby, Raab & McLean (2001) indicate that these contexts or learning opportunities should be "interesting and engaging and provide the child with contexts for exploring, practicing, and perfecting competence" (p. 90). When the early interventionist determines these contexts it is critical that the child and family's cultural background be taken into consideration.

When considering the appropriateness to the family, the early interventionist should provide services that treat families with dignity and respect and are sensitive to family cultural and socioeconomic diversity (Hanson & Bruder, 2001). Thus when the early interventionist focuses on the family, he or she should understand the family's rituals and routines. Maloney (2000) indicated that "ritual pervades society and culture and society's values and norms are expressed and transmitted through ritual" (p. 144). Schuck and Bucy (1997) indicated that, although families differ in socioeconomic status, ethnic background, and religious orientation, there are three types of rituals that are probably universal to all families. These include family celebrations (religious, secular holidays, and rites of passage), family traditions (vacations, birthday or anniversary customs), and daily rituals (patterned family interactions, such as mealtime customs and bedtime practices). Family rituals (including daily rituals) are "repetitious, highly valued, meaningful family activities that transmit the family's enduring values and attitudes" (Schuck & Bucy, 1997), whereas daily routines are observable and repetitious family behaviors that are important in structuring family life and that must be completed. Routines "lack the symbolic content and the compelling, anticipatory nature that rituals possess" (Schuck & Bucy, 1997). Maloney (2000) indicated that individuals learn from their participation in rituals. Jennings (1982) suggested that rituals are not senseless activities but are one way in which human beings make sense of their world and discover who they are in the world. Boyce, Jensen, James, and Peacock (1983) indicated that when a family has a set of stable, valued routines the family "is able to foster a sense of permanence and continuity among its members" (p. 198). Thus it is important for the early interventionist to identify the family routines (rituals) and facilitate the child's participation in them.

Early interventionists can gain insight into family rituals and routines through interviews and observation. Using both family rituals and family routines in intervention is important because "developmental interventions that fit easily into family rituals are more likely to be practiced" (Schuck & Bucy, 1997, p. 489). This information can be obtained from families through observation and interview.

Natural contexts or learning opportunities are the focus of early intervention services because not only are they family centered and built on the family's interactive patterns as denoted by their rituals and routines, but they also are the context in which children learn. Children requiring early intervention services must learn skills and behaviors through high-frequency, naturally occurring activities in their environment to increase the likelihood that generalization will occur. Generalization is the "ability to respond appropriately in unrehearsed conditions including the transfer of appropriate responses across persons, objects, materials, natural consequences, stimuli and time" (Sheldon & Rush, 2001, p. 3).

The early interventionist should always think about the age of the child and the developmental level of the learning environments. When the early interventionist thinks in terms of age and developmentally appropriate activities, he or she realizes that the interactions between caregivers and infants or toddlers change over time, as do the activities in which they engage. Neonates and young infants engage in a "bimodal system of environmental attention and interaction" (Noonan & McCormick, 1992, p. 149). As a child gets older, age and developmentally appropriate activities stress a "wider range of environmental interaction and control behaviors" (p. 149). Finally, the toddler or preschooler becomes increasingly interested in "family or home routines and the play of other children" (p. 149).

Dunst, Bruder, et al. (2001) indicated that learning opportunities that are interesting and engaging, competence producing, and mastery oriented are associated with optimal child learning. In another study, Dunst, Hamby, Trivette, Raab, and Bruder (2000) identified 22 categories of activity settings (learning opportunities) that they believe provide a framework for identifying competence-enhancing learning experiences that are family centered and have the characteristics that facilitate learning listed previously. Dunst, Bruder, et al. (2001) defined an activity setting as "a situation-specific experience, opportunity, or event that involves a child's interaction with people, the physical environment, or both, and provides a context for a child to learn about his or her own abilities and capabilities as well as the propensities and proclivities of others" (p. 70). These learning opportunities are a "mix of planned and unplanned, structured and unstructured, and intention and serendipitous life experiences" (Dunst, Trivette, et al., 2001, p. 50). The 22 categories of learning settings included family activity settings and community learning settings (Box 5-1). Focusing on the context or event in which intervention will take place is ecologically valid in that it references the child's current environments with an eye to future environments.

| Box 5-1 | *Family activity and community learning settings* |

Family Activity Settings
- A mix of adult activities in which a child becomes a participant (family routines, gardening activities)
- Activities exposing a child to daily chores (parenting activities)
- Activities enabling child acquisition of social-adaptive competencies (child activities)
- Activities bringing children in contact with other children and adults (socialization activities)
- Activities having special family meaning (family rituals and celebrations)
- Activities providing children with opportunities to practice emerging capabilities and learn new competencies (physical play and literacy activities), and
- Activities providing a context for expressing interest-based child abilities (play and entertainment activities)

Community Learning Settings
- Children's learning opportunities afforded through adult-oriented activities (outdoor activities)
- Family-oriented activities (family excursions and outings), child-oriented activities (play activities)
- Activities that bring children in contact with other children and adults (organizations or groups and church-related activities)
- Activities that include structured (arts or entertainment activities) as well as unstructured (children's attractions) learning experiences
- Activities that involve children in events that are culturally meaningful and community enmeshing (community activities), and
- Activities that involve other children of varying skill levels (recreation and sports activities)

From Dunst, C. J., Hamby, D., Trivette, C., Raab, M., & Bruder, M.B. (2000). Everyday family and community life and children's naturally occurring learning opportunities. *Journal of Early Intervention, 23*(3), 151-164.

Interventionists should take into consideration the characteristics of the events in which intervention takes place. These include whether the activity is child initiated or directed, and the event or activity structure. It is important to know if the activity is child initiated or directed because carryover of skills learned in activities that are initiated by the child has been found to be higher (Kellegrew, 1998). A description of the event or activity structure is crucial because the interventionist needs to know if the event is predictable (includes turn taking and multiple natural opportunities) in order to replicate the desired intervention outcome. Predictable events are important for learning in that they help the child make sense of the activity and the behavior that is the target of intervention. The event structure should naturally facilitate turn taking to allow the child to learn the conversational rules. The predictability of the events leads to an understanding that the repetition of the events is an important factor in learning. Bronfenbrenner (1999) indicated that "to be effective, activity must take place on a regular basis over an extended period of time" (p. 6). Predictability of events also lends itself to the use of scripted events. The use of scripts in intervention has been found to increase both socialization and language skills (Neeley, Neeley, Justen, and Tipton-Sumner, 2001).

Other important event characteristics include whether the event is planned or unplanned, includes other individuals, and is culturally meaningful. Planned and unplanned events are both part of the natural experiences of young children, and both types of events can provide the child with learning opportunities (Dunst et al., 2000). A planned learning opportunity can include the parent and child going to a regularly scheduled parent–child play group. Unplanned learning opportunities include such things as picking a flower and smelling it on a neighborhood walk. Unplanned learning opportunities are often overlooked, and the early interventionist should realize that learning is likely to take place whenever people interact.

Involvement of other individuals is crucial for social interaction and learning. Dunst et al. (2000) indicated that learning opportunities are those that involve participation in events as part of family and community life that do not necessarily include other children. These authors went on to say that "inclusion experiences and opportunities need to be considered as only one kind of natural learning environment" (p. 161). Families in general, and specifically families of children from culturally diverse backgrounds, are the only vehicles that can inform the early interventionist if the events targeted are meaningful to the child and are consistent with the child's environment, the family's behavior preferences, and the family's lifestyle (Davis-McFarland & Dowell, 2000).

Within these natural contexts the interventionist must determine the type of intervention procedures used. Hepting and Goldstein (1996) explained that naturalness of the intervention context seems independent of naturalness of intervention procedures. In their review of intervention studies, Hepting and Goldstein (1996) found that the procedures used in natural contexts range from adult-directed procedures to child-directed procedures and that both types of strategies are used in typical parent–child interactions. Adult-directed procedures can be found in the interactions between adults and typical children; these interactions usually focus on controlling child behaviors (Sachs, 2001). Child-directed intervention procedures are those that focus on facilitating the child's behavior and are also found in the natural interactions between adults and typical children. The early interventionist needs to take into account the "parenting styles and instructional practices characterized by contingent responsiveness to child-initiated and child-directed behavior and caregiver behavior that provides opportunities for practicing emerging skills and elaborating on existing capabilities" (Dunst, 2000, p. 102) when planning intervention to facilitate the child's communicative competence. One aspect of typical adult–child interactions is the use of a responsive style by the caregiver. Research has shown that a highly responsive style fosters communication (Warren, 2000; Yoder, Warren, McCathren, & Leew, 1998). A responsive style includes "such natural teaching devices as expansions; models; growth recasts; use of concrete, simplified vocabulary; talk about objects and events the child is attending to; and so forth, all finely tuned to the child's comprehension level" (Warren, 2000, p. 34). This responsive interactive style should be implemented by parents and all early intervention professionals. Warren (2000) suggested that "all responsible parties provide the most responsive and developmentally progressive learning environment possible for as many of the child's waking hours as possible" (p. 36). Thus the issue of the context in which intervention is provided and the techniques used by all involved in early intervention must be considered as a whole and not as separate parts of the process. Dunst, Trivette, et al. (2001) indicated that "contextually based child- initiated, and adult-directed learning opportunities provided by parents and mediated by practitioners have been used as natural learning opportunities for positively influencing child behavior and development" (p. 57). Dunst, Trivette, et al. (2001) further suggest that a mix of learning environments may be better than a "preponderance of only one type of practice."

Likewise, it is important to take into consideration the family's cultural interaction patterns when determining natural events for intervention and natural intervention procedures. More information on intervention techniques will be presented in Chapters 6 and 7.

Once the place where the intervention will take place has been determined, the interventionist should manipulate the environment to facilitate the child's participation in the event. The interventionist wants to increase the probability that the child will initiate communicative interaction through use of the targeted communication outcome. Event manipulation may occur in the structure of the event or in adaptation or manipulation of the materials used in the environment. Event manipulation may focus on changing or modifying the event structure so that the targeted outcome occurs repeatedly and is clear to the child. The interventionist should think through the physical dimension of the environment so that the amount of stimulation is appropriate to the child (Donahue-Kilburg, 1992). Another benefit of adapting the environment so that the targeted outcome occurs repeatedly is that the communicative environment can be loaded with models of the target behavior through caregiver or interventionist's use of self-talk, parallel talk, or both. However, as noted elsewhere in this chapter, the use of these language modeling techniques should be appropriate and in response to the child's focus or communicative behavior. Adaptation of the physical design and materials used within the event should facilitate the child's participation in the event. The early interventionist should determine the appropriate amount of stimuli. The environment should include familiar and comforting elements, as well as novelties to promote growth; it also should be warm and accepting to encourage interaction. Environmental manipulation should not violate the naturalness of the interaction. Adults in the environment should be attentive and responsive to the child.

Another issue to consider in the structure of the natural event is the caregiver's participation in the event and how he or she structures the event to allow child participation. One concept that is discussed in the literature on interactions between caregivers and typical children is that the caregiver should scaffold the event (Bruner, 1983). The caregiver introduces the interactive event in such a way that the caregiver is supporting the child's initial participation in the event; in fact, the caregiver is facilitating the whole event. As the child gains competence and experience, the caregiver removes some of the support provided to the child to facilitate interaction. Gradually, the child learns the interaction expectations of the event and becomes a full participant. It should be noted that "providing therapy in natural environments and using a child's play situations and daily routines does not just naturally happen. Parents must share their family stories, routines, and traditions, and all early intervention specialists must find creative ways to translate their expertise to design meaningful interventions with caregivers" (Hanft & Pilkington, 2000, p. 11).

In summary, the context of early intervention is an important concern for early interventionists. Natural environments or learning settings must be expanded to include all learning opportunities that can and do occur throughout the day and in all child environments. Hanson and Bruder (2001) indicated that "program administrators should ensure that interventions are designed to be delivered in the places where families spend time, or in places where families would like to spend time (grandmother's house, child care, exercise group, and so on)" (p. 52).

INDIVIDUAL FAMILY SERVICE PLANS

Part C of the Amendments to the Individuals with Disability Education Act (IDEA, P.L. 105-17, 1997) mandates that early intervention services for children aged 0 to 2 years be individualized and family-centered and include the development of the individualized family service plan (IFSP). For children between 3 and 5 years, an individualized education plan (IEP) should be implemented. IFSPs are family centered and should include a description of family resources, priorities, and concerns related to the child's development as associated with the family's desired outcomes. The IFSP should be derived from the family's concerns, priorities, and resources, as well as from a determination of the child's abilities. The IFSP should include a list of services (specifying the desired child/infant response), intervention strategies, activities, and person(s) responsible. Dunst (2000) indicated that family-centered practices must take into consideration child learning opportunities and parenting supports, as well as family and community resources and supports; thus, the IFSP must include this information. Fewell, Snyder, Sexton, Bertrand, and Hockless (1991) and Paul (2001) described seven elements that should be included in the IFSP. These are as follows:

- Information about the child's present level of physical, cognitive, social, emotional, communicative, and adaptive development.
- Information about the family's resources, priorities, and concerns.
- Outcome statements.
- Specific early intervention services to be provided to meet the needs of the child and the family.
- Dates for initiation and duration of services.
- Identification of service coordinator.
- Steps to be taken to support the child's transition to other services.

The IFSP may also include information about the child's physical positioning, material arrangements, or both (Noonan & McCormick, 1992). The above discussion noted the importance of environmental manipulation as well.

Another important function of the IFSP is to outline an evaluation system that can identify change, determine if generalization has occurred, and suggest any modification(s) that may be needed. It is necessary to identify change in a child for many reasons. "Teachers want to know if their intervention services and supports are helping children change. Parents want to know if their children are progressing. Administrators, evaluators, funding agencies, and policymakers want to know if programs produce change" (McConnell, 2000, p. 45). Data are also needed to determine if the child increases his or her use of the intervention outcomes in day-to-day interactions (generalization). The use of natural intervention contexts has been shown to be supportive, but data are needed to show that the child uses the outcomes in contexts other than those specified in the IFSP. Last, but of paramount importance, is that any data are collected should be used to modify IFSP outcomes. It is through the evaluation process that the IFSP can be made into a living document to meet current circumstances.

McWilliam, Ferguson, Harbin, Porter, Munn & Vandiviere (1998) indicated that the IFSP should be family centered so that the family is more in control. To be more in control the family needs to understand the major document pertaining to their early intervention services. Services should be family centered so as to support families as the constant caregivers for their child and as the primary influence on their child's development. McWilliam et al. (1998) indicated that families need a sense of control over decision making. Since the IFSP guides services, it must reflect family priorities and practices. Development of an IFSP is a process, and families want the process to be informal (Summers, Dell'Oliver, Turnbull, Benson, Santelli, Campbell & Spiegel-Causey, 1990). They also want the plan to be flexible (Able-Boone, Sandall, Loughry, & Frederick, 1990). McWilliam (1996b) presented the following list of useful characteristics for IFSP planning:

- Parents understand and agree with the content.
- Parents have a sense of ownership of the plan.
- The plan includes goals that are important to the family.
- Activities for accomplishing goals are enjoyable for the child and the family.
- Activities are embedded in daily routines.
- There is a high likelihood that goals can be accomplished in a relatively short time.
- Resources are available and accessible for implementing activities.
- The intervention plan is amenable to frequent changes and updating.
- The plan is reviewed frequently, and planning is a continuous process.
- The plan is written in the parent's language.

As a result of the early-intervention plan and action, parents "should attribute positive changes in their child's development and social–emotional adjustment" to their involvement in the intervention process (Mahoney & Wheeden, 1997).

One of the critical aspects of the IFSP is that it encompasses family and professional consensus on outcomes and natural contexts in which intervention should take place. There is a need to attune the professionals' expertise to the family's concerns. Gallagher and Desimone (1995) suggested that the role of the early interventionist is to provide expert advice and the family's role is to make the decisions.

Eiserman, Weber, and McCoun (1995) indicated that the varied roles that professionals and parents may have to assume while providing early intervention services are in flux. The roles of the early interventionist are diverse during the intervention process. Roles may include that of advisor, counselor, and supplier of information to families, in addition to the more traditional role of direct care provider. However, interventionists usually assist parents in making choices about their role in intervention and help them to develop the skills they need to provide direct intervention with their child. In addition, interventionists may provide direct services to the child. One caution should be stated at this point: early interventionists need to learn that their personal preferences or comfort in providing direct intervention to the child or direct intervention with the caregiver should not dictate the intervention program. Thus it is important that the early interventionist be supportive and nonjudgmental, recognize that the family is the ultimate decision maker, and be accepting of families' social and cultural diversity (Gallagher & Desimone, 1995, p. 368). Hanft and Pilkington (2000) suggested that interventionists implement five strategies for developing early intervention and in so doing determine their role in the process. Hanft and Pilkington's strategies include the following:

- Help families articulate priorities.
- Prioritize meaningful function practical outcomes.
- Consider, experience, and support the variety of environments and adult caregivers who interact with the child.
- Use flexible service delivery models.
- Ensure ongoing and frequent evaluation of whether therapy makes a difference.

The roles that parents assume in early intervention have tended toward direct involvement in service provision. More specifically, the family's and caregiver's role includes the implementation of appropriate intervention strategies (with adequate support from the early interventionist). Yet the interventionist must realize that not all families are ready or able to assume this role initially. Families must be informed of the options they have in the intervention process. In fact, families want professionals to relay information about their child and the services that are available, but they ultimately want to be empowered to make informed decisions (Able-Boone et al., 1990). Early interventionists must realize that each family is a unique system; thus the role assumed by any specific family or family member will vary based on how the family's culture affects their participation and communication (Gallagher & Desimone, 1995), as well as the family's comfort level with the early intervention process.

Eiserman et al. (1995) conducted a study comparing an early intervention program where the professionals provided direct intervention services with a program that focused on training parents (mothers) to use therapeutic techniques. At a follow-up 42 months after the initiation of intervention, reassessment findings indicated that children in both groups performed equally well. However, parents preferred direct involvement and responsibility in addressing their child's developmental needs. These authors suggested that providing families with options about the roles that parents and professionals assume in an early intervention program is important.

GUIDELINES FOR EFFECTIVE HOME VISITS

The goal of home visits is to establish an optimal and effective learning situation that allows both the infant or toddler and the caregiver to develop active rather than passive roles in the early intervention program (Davis-McFarland & Dowell, 2000). Early interventionists must always remember that the home is the family's dominion and that they are guests. The early interventionist should remember not to make any assumptions about the family's concerns, priorities, and resources upon entering the home. When beginning the home visit it is essential to develop rapport with the family and to use an interactive style that fosters an atmosphere of warmth and sincerity. Hershberger (1991) indicated that the early interventionist should allow time for the caregivers to discuss any changes since the last visit. Listening to parents or caregivers lets them know how important they are to the early intervention process and allows the parents or caregivers to have an active role in mapping out the course of the intervention program. Hershberger (1991) also indicated that the early interventionist should observe not only the interactive and nurturing style of the caregivers but also the physical environment of the home (e.g., where the toys are and where the family congregates). A final reminder for the early interventionist upon initiating home visits is that families are concerned about the intrusiveness of the intervention and their privacy.

BUILDING SUPPORT NETWORKS

An essential aspect of providing family-centered early intervention is that the early interventionist needs to focus "on a range of informal community resources as sources of parenting and family supports" (Hanson & Bruder, 2001). Thus during intervention, support networks should be built. The early interventionist is part of the support network, but access to resources in the larger community should be developed. One of the roles of the early interventionist is to know what types of services are available in his or her community and to share that knowledge with the family. Dunst (2000) indicated that "family and community supports include any number and type of intrafamily, informal, community and formal resources needed by parents to have the time and energy to engage in parenting and child-rearing activities" (p. 102). McWilliam (1996b) indicated that the family probably had some sort of support network before the beginning of early intervention services. McWilliam (1996b) also indicated that the interventionists should not "supplant existing sources of support, make families overly dependent on us, and should not allow a situation to occur in which a family leaves our services without a system of support in place and the skills and knowledge to use the resources available to them" (pp. 138-139). A truly family-centered approach to early intervention "allows families to gain a sense of control over their lives while strengthening their existing internal and external supports" (Able-Boone et al., 1990, p. 111) as well as creating new external supports. Parent support networks influence parenting "by providing emotional and instrumental support, encouraging or discouraging specific parenting attitudes and behaviors and providing models and opportunities to learn alternative or new parenting and childrearing interactional styles" (Dunst, 2001, p. 102). Parent support networks influence the parenting style, and this has an impact on child behavior and development.

REFERENCES

Able-Boone, H., Sandall, S. R., Loughry, A., & Frederick, L. L. (1990). An informed, family-centered approach to Public Law 99-457: Parental views. *Topics in Early Childhood Special Education, 10*(1), 100-111.

Boyce, W. T., Jensen, E. W., James, S. A., & Peacock, J. L. (1983). The family routine inventory: Theoretical origins. *Social Science and Medicine, 17*(4), 193-200.

Bronfenbrenner, U. (1999). Environments in developmental perspectives. Theoretical and operational models. In S. L. Friedman & T. D. Wachs (Eds.), *Measuring environment across the life span: Emerging methods and concepts* (pp. 3-28). Washington, DC: American Psychological Association.

Bruder, M. B., & Dunst, C. J. (2000). Expanding learning opportunities for infants and toddlers in natural environments. *Zero to Three, 20*(2), 34-36.

Bruner, J. (1983). *Child's talk: Learning to use language.* New York: Norton.

Davis-McFarland, E., & Dowell, B. (2000). Sociocultural issues in assessment and intervention. In L. Watson, E. Crais, & T. Layton (Eds.), *Handbook of early language impairment in children: Assessment and treatment* (pp. 73-109). Albany, NY: Delmar Thomson Learning.

Donahue-Kilburg, G. (1992). *Family-centered early intervention for communication disorders: Prevention and treatment.* Gaithersburg, MD: Aspen.

Dunst, C. J. (2000). Revisiting "Rethinking Early Intervention." *Topics in Early Childhood Special Education, 20*(2), 95-104.

Dunst, C. J., Bruder, M. B., Trivette, C., Hamby, D., Raab, M., & McLean, M. (2001). Characteristics and consequences of everyday natural learning opportunities. *Topics in Early Childhood Special Education, 21*(2), 68-92.

Dunst, C. J., Hamby, D., Trivette, C., Raab, M., & Bruder, M. B. (2000). Everyday family and community life and children's naturally occurring learning opportunities. *Journal of Early Intervention, 23*(3), 151-164.

Dunst, C. J., Trivette, C. M., Humphries, T., Raab, M., & Roper, N. (2001). Contrasting approaches to natural learning environments interventions. *Infants and Young Children, 14*(2), 48-63.

Eiserman, W. D., Weber, C., & McCoun, M. (1995). Parent and professional roles in early intervention: A longitudinal comparison of the effects of two intervention configurations. *Journal of Special Education, 29*(1), 20-44.

Fewell, R. R., Snyder, P., Sexton, D., Bertrand, S., & Hockless, M. F. (1991). Implementing IFSPs in Louisiana: Different formats for family-centered practices under Part H. *Topics in Early Childhood Special Education, 11*(3), 54-65.

Gallagher, J., & Desimone, L. (1995). Lessons learned from implementation of the IEP: Applications to the IFSP. *Topics in Early Childhood Special Education, 15*(3), 351-378.

Hanft, B. E., & Pilkington, K. O. (2000). Therapy in natural environments: The means or end goal for early intervention? *Infants and Young Children, 12*(4), 1-13.

Hanson, M. J., & Bruder, M. B. (2001). Early intervention: Promises to keep. *Infants and Young Children, 13*(3), 47-58.

Hepting, N. H., & Goldstein, H. (1996). What's natural about naturalistic language intervention? *Journal of Early Intervention, 20*(2), 249-265.

Hershberger, P. (1991). A naturalistic approach to home-based early intervention. *Infant-Toddler Intervention: The Transdisciplinary Journal, 1*(2), 83-92.

Individuals with Disabilities Education Act Amendments of 1997 [U.S. Code of Federal Regulations 303.12(4)(b)(2)].

Jennings, T. W. (1982). On ritual knowledge. *The Journal of Religion, 62*(2), 111-127.

Kellegrew, D.,H. (1998) Creating opportunities for occupation: An intervention to promote self-care independence of young children with special needs. *American Journal of Occupational Therapy, 52,* 457-465.

Mahoney, G., & Wheeden, C. A. (1997). Parent–child interaction—The foundation for family-centered early intervention practice: A response to Baird and Peterson. *Topics in Early Childhood Special Education, 17*(2), 165-187.

Maloney, C. (2000). The role of ritual in preschool settings. *Early Childhood Education Journal, 27*(3), 143-150.

McConnell, S. R. (2000). Assessment in early intervention and early childhood special education: Building on the past to project into our future. *Topics in Early Childhood Special Education, 20*(1), 43-48.

McLean, J. (1989). A language-communication model. In D. Bernstein & E. Tiegerman (Eds.), *Language and communication disorders in children* (2nd Ed.) (pp. 208-228). Columbus, OH: Merrill.

McWilliam, P. J. (1996a). Day-to-day service provision. In P. J. McWilliam, P. J. Winton, & E. R. Crais (Eds.). *Practical strategies for family-centered intervention* (pp. 125-154*).* San Diego: Singular.

McWilliam, P. J. (1996b). Family-centered intervention planning. In P. J. McWilliam, P. J. Winton, & E. R. Crais (Eds.). *Practical strategies for family-centered intervention* (pp. 97-123*).* San Diego: Singular.

McWilliam, R. A., Ferguson, A., Harbin, G. L., Porter, P., Munn, D., & Vandiviere, P. (1998). The family-centeredness of individualized family service plans. *Topics in Early Childhood Special Education, 18*(2), 69-82.

Neeley, P. M., Neeley, R. A., Justen, J. E. III, & Tipton-Sumner, C. (2001). Scripted play as a language intervention strategy for preschoolers with developmental disabilities. *Early Childhood Special Education, 28*(4), 243-246.

Noonan, M. J., & McCormick, L. (1992). A naturalistic curriculum model for early intervention. *Infant-Toddler Intervention: The Transdisciplinary Journal, 2*(3), 147-159.

Owens, R. E. (1999). *Language disorders: A functional approach to assessment and intervention* (3rd Ed). Boston: Allyn & Bacon.

Paul, R. (2001). *Language disorders: From infancy through adolescence* (2nd Ed). St Louis, MO: Mosby.

Roper, N., & Dunst, C. J. (2003). Communication intervention in natural learning environments: Guidelines for practice. *Infants and Young Children, 16*(3), 215-226.

Sachs, J. (2001). Communication development in infancy. In Berko Gleason, J. (Ed.), *The development of language* (5th Ed). Boston: Allyn & Bacon.

Schuck, L. A., & Bucy, J. E. (1997). Family rituals: Implications for early intervention. *Topics in Early Childhood Special Education, 17*(4), 477-493.

Sheldon, M. L., & Rush, D. D. (2001). The ten myths about providing early intervention services in natural environments. *Infants and Young Children, 14*(1), 1-13.

Sparks, S. N. (1989). Assessment and intervention with at-risk infants and toddlers. Guidelines for the speech–language pathologist. *Topics in Language Disorders, 10*(1), 43-56.

Summers, J. A., Dell'Oliver, C., Turnbull, A., Benson, H., Santelli, E., Campbell M., & Spiegel-Causey, E. (1990). Examining the individualized family service plan process: What are family and practitioner preferences? *Topics in Early Childhood Special Education, 10*(1), 78-99.

Warren, S. F. (2000). The future of early communication and language intervention. *Topics in Early Childhood Special Education, 20*(1), 33-37.

Yoder, P. J., Warren, S. F., McCathren, R., & Leew, S. V. (1998). Does adult responsivity to child behavior facilitate communication development? In A. M. Wetherby, S. F. Warren, & J. Reichle (Eds.), *Transitions in prelinguistic communication* (pp.39-58). Baltimore: Brookes.

CHAPTER 6

Components of Speech–Language and Communication Intervention

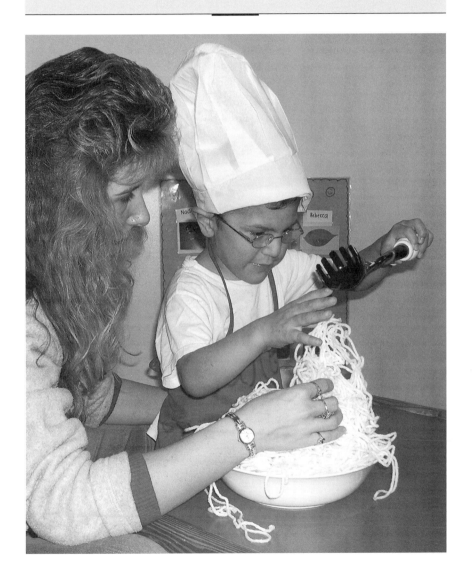

OUTLINE

This chapter discusses intervention that focuses on communication skills of the infant and young child and elaborates on the framework presented in Chapter 5, refining it so that it focuses on the speech–language pathologist's role in the early intervention process. Principles that should be incorporated into the intervention process to enhance the communication process are presented. Chapter 7 focuses on parents' involvement in the intervention process, and Chapter 8 presents the case studies, this time focusing on the intervention program.

THE FIVE QUESTIONS OF INTERVENTION

A model for intervention should take into consideration many factors that have an impact on the provision of communication intervention services. The following are some aspects that must be considered (adapted from Owens, 1999; Weiss, 2001):

- Language facilitator: Who?
- Natural language: Why?
- General intervention guidelines: What?
- Contextual influence on communication: Where?
- Intervention procedures: How?

Who Will Be the Language Facilitator?

The facilitator should be someone with whom the child wants to communicate. Early intervention practices tell us that often the communication facilitator is a family member. As was mentioned in Chapter 5, young children are likely to be in activity settings that involve the home. When working with a family member, the speech–language pathologist is collaborating with that person, providing techniques and insights about how to facilitate language. MacDonald and Carroll (1992) indicated that every interaction a child is involved in presents an opportunity for that child to learn social and communication competence; therefore all early intervention professionals need to "fine-tune their communication with children." There may be times when the language facilitator is the speech–language pathologist who provides intervention services in a more direct approach, and there may be other times when the language facilitator is another member of the early intervention team, a caregiver, a peer, or a community representative. The most important concept to remember is that the language facilitator must be a sincere communication partner who conveys genuine messages.

Why Should Language or Communication Intervention Consider Natural Language?

Language or communication intervention should closely approximate the natural communication process because language is not learned in a vacuum but rather during dynamic interactions with responsive partners. Communication and language develop in a social context to achieve largely social ends (Carpenter, Nagell, & Tomasello, 1998). Communication occurs in natural contexts for naturally occurring reasons (intents). When working with young children, the early interventionist should remember to focus on communicative exchanges as they occur naturally in everyday environments. The major focus should be to provide the child with a communication system that is effective, efficient, and flexible.

What Should Be the Focus of Language or Communication Intervention?

The focus of communication intervention should be functional communication outcomes; the ultimate goal of intervention is age-appropriate communication. The outcomes should "enhance the child's ability to effectively communicate in a variety of settings" (Weiss, 2001, p. 102). The speech–language pathologist may follow developmental guidelines with a specific focus on language usage, form, and content. Nonverbal communicative means are the basis for communication, which implies that language function is acquired before language form. This means that children use the communication or language abilities they possess to accomplish some communicative goal. Owens (1999) suggested some principles that underlie the following developmental guidelines. These include the following:

- Language evolves from nonverbal communication.
- Social and cognitive prerequisites are necessary for the child to use language in certain ways.
- Simple rules are acquired before more difficult ones.
- Development is not uniform across all aspects of language.
- At different levels of development, children act differently (Owens, 1999, p. 249).

When the early interventionist determines intervention outcomes, many factors are taken into consideration. The first determination is based on the results of the assessment (including parent interview, report, and participation results; results of formal or structured methods; and results of informal measures or observations). A developmental approach might be used to determine what skill the infant or toddler next needs to learn in order to develop an effective communication system. A strengths-or-weaknesses approach is used to determine the child's strengths as opposed to areas that are in need of facilitation. The family's desired communication outcomes for the intervention services must also be determined. The professional information must be balanced with the family's desired outcomes for the intervention services. Input from the parent and caregiver about the relevance of specific communicative behaviors to the child and the family's life must be evaluated.

Paul (2001) indicated that when deciding on communication and language outcomes the child's "zone of proximal development" should also be considered in addition to a developmental approach. The zone of proximal development is the "distance between a child's current level of independent functioning and potential level of performance" (p. 65). When the zone of proximal development is used, it is considered a waste of the child's time if the interventionist chooses an outcome that the child already knows; teaching an outcome that is above the child's knowledge base would also be considered inefficient and probably unattainable for the child. Thus expanding on this framework, the outcomes of intervention will differ depending on whether the child is prelinguistic, early linguistic (emerging language), or linguistic (developing language).

Leonard (1992) suggested that intervention outcomes be based not only on the child's current communication status but also on an assessment of the child's communication styles and effectiveness as well as reported family concern. The intervention outcomes should enhance the child's functional communication with others, as well as foster development of communication skills. Leonard suggested that some general communication intervention outcomes might include the following:

- Increase the number of enjoyable and successful communications with family members.
- Increase the child's communicative attempts.
- Increase responsiveness to adult communication.
- Increase intelligible speech production.
- Increase the variety of content and forms (pp. 230-231).

Weiss (1997) suggested that no matter what approach the early interventionist uses to determine the outcomes of intervention, there are several questions that must be answered (Box 6-1).

Weiss (2001) indicated that there are two ways in which intervention can be provided, which also influence determination of the language or communication outcomes that are selected. One way in which intervention can be implemented is to provide general language stimulation. In this mode, overall language is encouraged. Weiss (2001) indicates that no specific language goals (outcomes) are delineated "other than enriching their (the child's) language-learning environment in all possible ways" (p. 118). Paul (2001) called this method of intervention "indirect language stimulation." She indicated that this method of language intervention provides the child with simple and accessible models of the language that maps the child's actions or intents and

---

| **Box 6-1** | *Questions to ask before implementing an intervention plan* |

- What presentation methods facilitate the child's ability to demonstrate new language targets?
- How much stimulus support does the child need to be successful?
- Is the child willing to risk being wrong?
- What motivates the child to improve language performance?
  (Weiss, 2001, p. 295)

the language form that could be used to express them. According to Weiss (2001), the other manner in which intervention can be implemented is by use of focused language stimulation techniques. In this technique, specific goals (outcomes) are selected for the child. The child is then "bombarded by the targeted form(s) or function(s) missing from the child's repertoire and the examples are presented frequently and in unambiguous contexts" (p. 118).

Where Should Language or Communication Intervention Take Place?

Language is influenced by context because language and communication abilities are based on an individual's social, cultural, and interpersonal competence. As discussed in Chapter 5, natural learning opportunities occur in the child's daily activity settings. In other words, a child does not typically request a toy during a snack event, but might request a food or drink item; thus knowledge of the snack event (e.g., a time to eat and drink) influences the way the child communicates and uses language (requests). Language learning is most efficient when the child can directly observe and experience the function and utility of the communication itself. Language intervention should occur within everyday events during the context of the give-and-take of conversation. Both the linguistic and nonlinguistic supports that could facilitate learning should be determined. The speech-language pathologist should ensure that when the child's everyday environments are used as the context for intervention, these settings also promote responsive language facilitator–child interactions. Warren, Yoder, and Leew (2002) indicated that because the environment should be one in which children can initiate communication about things they need, want, or find interesting, the interventionist might have to arrange the child's immediate environment to enhance communication. Warren et al. (2002) also indicated that communication opportunities arise when "the predictability and order of an environment is violated" (p. 131) and that the language facilitator can either plan these occurrences or make the most out of those that are unplanned.

How Should Intervention Proceed?

The types of intervention procedures that are employed when providing communication services to infants and young children are very important. The facilitation techniques should conform to what the child can understand; therefore the level of techniques should be just slightly more advanced than the child's level of output (Weiss, 2001). Infants and toddlers do not learn through drill and practice but through experiences in familiar environments. Therefore the language intervention techniques used with a child this age should be nurturant and naturalistic (Duchan & Weitzner-Lin, 1987). The nurturant aspects of the process require that the early interventionist follow the child's lead and employ child-centered techniques. The early interventionist should focus on what interests the child (Owens, 1999). Following the child's lead sustains the child's interest in the activities and in the social interaction or communication (Hepting & Goldstein, 1996).

When the early interventionist interacts with a young, communicatively impaired child, it is crucial that he or she respond to the child's communicative intent and action. The responses are considered nurturant because they facilitate language; the responses to the child are contingent upon what the child says or the communicative intent expressed by the child. These responses can generally be categorized as acceptance, modeling, and nonacceptance responses. Examples of these responses are shown in Box 6-2 (elaboration of Duchan & Weitzner-Lin, 1987).

The naturalistic aspects of the language intervention techniques employed refer to the events in which language is facilitated. The language facilitator must recognize the communication learning potential of naturally occurring activities. Chapter 5 presented a review of the influence of family routines and routine activities on learning. However, routines are only one type of event in which communication occurs. Duchan and Weitzner-Lin (1987) indicated that different types of events have their own unique characteristics and structure, which provide different communication opportunities for the child and should be incorporated into the intervention process (because the goal is to develop an effective, efficient, and flexible communication system). Some other types of events that the language facilitator can use to his or her advantage in facilitating language include scripts, stories (and other types of narratives), different types of play (manipulative or pretend play), games (or more structured play), and conversations.

Neeley, Neeley, Justen, and Tipton-Sumner (2001) and Goldstein and Cisar (1992) conducted studies in which they taught scripted play to preschool children with disabilities and found increases in social and communicative or

---

Box 6-2   *Acceptance, modeling, and nonacceptance responses*

Acceptance Responses
- Acknowledge or affirm
- Provide a nonverbal response
- Repeat what the child says
- Expand what the child says
- Extend what the child says
- Translate the child's unconventional acts
- Signal turn exchanged

Modeling Responses
- Translate the child's unconventional act (e.g., model what could be said in that context [using parallel talk, comments, labels, or requests])
- Expand the child's communicative message (rephrase)
- Extend the child's communicative message (e.g., add information that is relevant)
- Cue the child by providing a model for the child based on what the language facilitator assumes the child's intent would be (based on the characteristics of the event)
- Note that it is important that the modeled response provide the form needed to encode the child's communicative intent or act

Nonacceptance Responses
- Direct: the adult intentionally misunderstands the child
- Indirect: the adult subtly creates a communicative breakdown

verbal interactions. Neeley et al. (2001) suggested that scripted play is a useful intervention tool for increasing language and socialization in preschool children with disabilities.

Dale, Crain-Thoreson, Notari-Syverson, and Cole (1996) conducted a study of children with language delays in which parents were trained to provide interactive, responsive book reading. The study confirmed that joint book reading is a context in which language can be facilitated. Nelson (1998) indicated that early book reading is specifically useful for establishing joint attention and referencing, taking turns, and developing new vocabulary items. It also provides a context for interacting with print as a means of developing early literacy. It should be noted that narrative structure and parent interaction with books reflect the cultural identity of the family. For example, Anderson-Yockel and Haynes (1994) found that African American mothers and white mothers had many similarities when interacting with their toddlers in a joint book-reading event, but they also found differences in the use of questions.

Play is a context in which language intervention can take place. Play has been called child's work. It is a naturally occurring context in which manipulation of objects and materials can be functional, symbolic, or constructive. Hubbell (1981) indicated that facilitative play could be used to facilitate language. The interventionist arranges the activity so that within the play context the targeted outcomes occur naturally. According to Paul (2001), in facilitative play the child is in the driver's seat because the interventionist does not control the activity but rather follows the child's lead. Pretend play is an avenue in which the child's continued advances to represent events and meaning symbolically take place. As discussed earlier in this book, there seems to be a relationship between language and early symbolic play. Pretend play is only one type of play. Another type of play is playing games. Games are highly structured because there tends to be a specified turn assignment. Not only is the turn structure of games preplanned, but the content that can be uttered during a game is limited to that which is prescribed by the game itself. Although games may provide opportunities for repetition of specified outcomes, they tend to be highly controlled by the game-playing context.

Conversation is the major discourse format in which communication occurs. Conversations tend to be collaborative because each conversational partner contributes to a topic but is sensitive to whether or not the conversational partner understands the topic. Conversations are inclined to have somewhat formal opening and closing statements, be topic focused, and have a turn-taking structure.

Some event characteristics that must be examined when one determines the type of event in which the intervention will take place include the following:

- Is the event child initiated or adult directed?
- Is the event tightly or loosely structured?
- Does the event have predictable sequences or is it free flowing?
- Can the environment be manipulated so that the structure occurs repeatedly and is clear to the child, or is it part of a natural interaction that is unpredictable and cannot be manipulated?

- Can the event be scaffolded to provide the language learner with support (both linguistic and nonlinguistic), or is the event formalized?

CHILD-CENTERED INTERVENTION TECHNIQUES

Child-centered intervention techniques have been reported in the literature. When taught to caregivers, modifications of these techniques are often called interactive techniques. Interactive techniques can be considered as either interaction promoting or language facilitating. When used by the speech–language pathologist, the division is not as apparent because the goal of the speech–language pathologist is to facilitate language as well as to promote interaction. See Weiss (2001), Paul (2001), Owens (1999), Tannock and Girolametto (1992), and Duchan and Weitzner-Lin (1987) for more complete discussions of these techniques.

Expansion refers to elaboration of a child's utterance. The speech–language pathologist takes what the child says and fills in information to render the utterance grammatically correct. He or she adds grammatical markers and function words. For example, if the child says "cat" (while petting the family's sleeping cat), the adult might say, "The cat is sleeping." According to Weiss (2001), the purpose of an expansion is not only to acknowledge the child's attempt but also to provide an improved version of that attempt.

Extensions, sometimes called *expatiations*, are comments that add information to the child's communicative attempt. An expansion makes the child's communication grammatically correct, whereas an extension adds information, usually semantic, to the child's utterance. Owens (1999) indicated that an "extension is a reply to the content of the child's utterance that provides additional information on the topic" (p. 279).

Imitation is repetition of the child's utterance without changing the form (expansion) or adding content (extension). The adult's imitation involves either the child's whole utterance or part of it. Imitation has been used in numerous ways. One way to use imitation is to repeat the child's utterance without evaluation to show the child that his or her utterance was acceptable. Weiss (1997) indicated that the adult's imitating the child without evaluation can also serve to maintain the conversational topic by "letting the child know that the clinician acknowledges the topic established by the child" (p. 302). Another way in which imitation has been used is to provide the child with a correct model of speech and language with the expectation that the child will reimitate the adult's model. When the child repeats the adult language it is hoped that he or she will acquire some aspect of the adult's correct form. Imitation as a response as described above is different from elicited imitation. Elicited imitation occurs when the interventionist asks the child to imitate a language form. Lund and Duchan (1993) indicated that elicited imitation is unnatural because in natural conversation one is rarely asked to repeat what another person says.

Modeling is a "procedure in which the speech–language pathologist produces a rule-governed utterance at appropriate junctures in conversation or activities but does not ask the child to imitate" (Owens, 1999, p. 275). The adult's utterances are appropriate to the situation and are an attempt by the speech–language pathologist to provide the child with an utterance that is appropriate for expressing the content of the interaction. Modeling can also be used to provide the words to code the child's wants, feelings, and intended messages, in which case the speech–language pathologist is employing parallel talk. In parallel talk the speech–language pathologist may also talk about what the child is doing. Modeling can also be used in a self-talk fashion, in which the speech–language pathologist talks about what he or she is doing. Another type of modeling is focused stimulation. In this type of modeling a key word or phrase is repeated for emphasis. Fey, Cleave, Long, and Hughes (1993) indicated that focused stimulation should be semantically and pragmatically appropriate. Weiss (2001) indicated that when the speech–language pathologist uses modeling the long-term goal "may be to increase the child's production of relevant utterances, increase the child's use of a diverse lexicon, or increase conversational turn length" (p. 121).

Buildup and *breakdown* involve segmenting the child's utterance into shorter units and recombining the units to show the child how language goes together. Specifically, in breakdowns the child's utterance is repeated by building it up in grammatical form; then it is broken down into "several phrase-sized pieces in a series of sequential utterances that overlap in content" (Paul, 2001, p. 71). In a buildup the speech–language pathologist presents a sequence of phrase-sized units that when combined provide a more complete expression of the child's intended meaning.

Recast sentences change the child's utterances by changing the sentence type. The child's original intent of the message is not changed, nor is the content (semantics) changed. Owens (1999) indicated that recasts could be in the language form that the speech–language pathologist has targeted for intervention but suggested that this technique is easier to use in comment form than in question form. Nelson, Camarata, Welsh, Butkovsky, and Camarata (1996) found that conversational recasts are facilitated acquisition of targeted grammatical forms.

The speech–language pathologist also should remember that communication takes place in an interaction and that interactions have communicative turns. Therefore the speech–language pathologist should encourage the child to take another turn in the communicative interaction. Specific child-centered techniques that encourage the child to take another turn include turnabouts, back channels, balancing, and matching.

Turnabouts are a conversational approach in which the language facilitator acknowledges the child's utterance and then either asks for more information or makes a comment. Duchan and Weitzner-Lin (1987) indicated that the acceptance includes new information. MacDonald and Gilette (1984) indicated that turnabouts prevent dead-end contracts, which are exchanges that end after two turns.

Back channels are more indirect responses to children that acknowledge the child's communicative turn or encourage the child to continue (head nod, repeat, "uh-huh").

Balancing refers to adult–child interactions in which neither partner assumes control (MacDonald and Carroll, 1992). Balanced exchanges are "reciprocal in that each person influences the other" (p. 24). A key strategy that the language facilitator can use to create a more balanced interaction and thus encourage the child to respond is to wait expectantly for the child to take his or her turn. A complement to waiting expectantly is to give the child enough time to respond.

Matching "refers to the style in which a more advanced person acts and communicates in ways the less developed person (often the infant or young child) can perform and in ways that relate meaningfully to the child's immediate experiences" (MacDonald & Carroll, 1992, p. 25). In other words, the language facilitator responds to the child by using behaviors that are in the child's repertoire and are not beyond the child's interests and abilities.

More clinician-focused intervention procedures are presented in the literature. These intervention techniques are not detailed here because it is believed that young children learn best through natural experiences. Clinician-focused strategies can include drill and practice, drill play, elicited imitation, patterned elicitations, and direct questioning. See Paul (2001) and Owens (1999) for a review of these more direct intervention approaches. Such approaches have been criticized as not being naturalistic because the clinician is asking the child to engage in "communicative" exchanges that are not rooted in real life and do not resemble the world outside the intervention setting (Fey, 1986; Lund & Duchan, 1993).

When compared with the child-centered intervention techniques and the more direct clinician-focused approaches, a different group of language intervention techniques have been called hybrid approaches (Fey, 1986, Paul, 2001). These approaches fall in the middle of a continuum of naturalness (Fey, 1986). Included in these hybrid approaches are milieu teaching (mand-model or incidental teaching format) and script therapy. For information on the milieu approach, see Hart and Risley (1975) and Warren and Kaiser (1986); for information on incidental teaching and on the mand-model, consult Rogers-Warren and Warren (1985). These hybrid approaches are considered to be at the midpoint of the naturalness continuum because the context of developing language is naturalistic and the facilitator establishes joint attention with the child. However, such approaches also incorporate more direct techniques because the language facilitator requests that the child talk (a more direct technique). Script therapy is based on the use of joint action routines that have been scripted and on the violation of these routines. This theory is hybrid because the scripts are based on real-life events and directive because the violations are demands for performance (elicited imitation). For more information on script therapy, see Olswang and Bain (1991).

FAMILY-CENTERED PRACTICES

As presented in Chapter 5, intervention with young children who have communicative impairments should be family focused. The natural setting and the routine activities of the home provide the most appropriate context in which to do intervention because they are the most meaningful. Likewise, the most significant communicator is one who communicates for real purposes (e.g., the caregiver). Family-centered practices enlist the caregivers to participate in the intervention program, and the fact that the home setting is most natural increases the probability that the child will generalize the language being facilitated. However, not "every family is willing and/or able to participate in a family-centered approach. Without being judgmental, early interventionists need to determine the degree to which the family is willing to participate" (Weiss, 2001, p. 109) in the intervention program. When a family is not actively involved in the treatment the speech–language pathologist must employ the above-described child-centered intervention techniques.

REFERENCES

Anderson-Yockel, J., & Haynes, W. O. (1994). Joint book-reading strategies in working class African American and white mother–toddler dyads. *Journal of Speech and Hearing Research, 37*(3), 583-593.

Carpenter, M., Nagell, K., & Tomasello, M. (1998). Social cognition, joint attention, and communicative competency from 9 to 15 months of age. *Monographs of the Society for Research in Child Development, 63* (Serial No. 4).

Dale, P. S., Crain-Thoreson, C., Notari-Syverson, A., & Cole, K. (1996). Parent–child book reading as an intervention technique for young children with language delays. *Topics in Early Childhood Special Education, 16*(2), 213-235.

Duchan, J., & Weitzner-Lin, B. (1987). Nurturant-naturalistic intervention for language-impaired children: Implications for planning lessons and tracking progress. *ASHA,* July, 45-48.

Fey, M. (1986). *Language intervention with young children.* Needham Heights, MA: Allyn & Bacon.

Fey, M. E., Cleave, P. L., Long, S. H., & Hughes, D. L. (1993). Two approaches to the facilitation of grammar in children with language impairment: An experimental evaluation. *Journal of Speech and Hearing Research, 27,*141-157.

Goldstein, H., & Cisar, C. (1992). Promoting interaction during socio-dramatic play: Teaching scripts to typical preschoolers and classmates with disabilities. *Journal of Experimental Analysis of Behavior, 25*, 265-280.

Hart, B., & Risley, T. (1975). Incidental teaching of language in the preschool. *Journal of Applied Behavior Analysis, 813*, 411-420.

Hepting, H. H., & Goldstein, H. (1996). What's natural about naturalistic language intervention? *Journal of Early Intervention, 20*, 250-278.

Hubbell, R. (1981). *Children's language disorders: An integrated approach.* Englewood Cliffs, NJ: Prentice Hall.

Leonard, J. S. (1992). Communication intervention for young children at risk for specific communication disorders. *Seminars in Speech and Language, 13*(3), 223-236.

Lund, N., & Duchan, J. (1993). Assessing children's language in naturalistic contexts (3rd Ed.). Englewood Cliffs, NJ: Prentice Hall.

MacDonald, J., & Carroll J. (1992). A partnership for communicating with infants at risk. *Infants and Young Children, 4*(3), 20-30.

MacDonald, J., & Gilette, Y. (1984). Conversation engineering: A pragmatic approach to early social competence. *Seminars in Speech and Language, 5*, 171-183.

Neeley, P. M., Neeley, R. A., Justen, J. E. III, & Tipton-Sumner, C. (2001). Scripted play as a language intervention strategy for preschoolers with developmental disabilities. *Early Childhood Special Education, 28*(4), 243-246.

Nelson, N. W. (1998). *Childhood language disorders in context: Infancy through adolescence* (2nd Ed). Boston: Allyn & Bacon.

Nelson, K., Camarata, S. M., Welsh, J. Butkovsky, L., & Camarata, M. (1996). Effects of imitative and conversational recasting treatment on the acquisition of grammar in children with specific language impairment and younger language-normal children. *Journal of Speech and Hearing Disorders, 39*(4), 850-859.

Olswang, L., & Bain, B. (1991). Intervention issues for toddlers with specific language impairments. *Topics in Language Disorders, 11*, 69-86.

Owens, R. (1999) *Language disorders: A functional approach to assessment and intervention,* (3rd Ed). Boston: Allyn & Bacon.

Paul, R. (2001). *Language disorders from infancy through adolescence: Assessment and intervention* (2nd Ed). St Louis, MO: Mosby.

Rogers-Warren, A., & Warren, S. (1985). Mands for verbalization: Facilitating the display of newly trained language in children. *Behavior Modification, 4*, 230-245.

Tannock, R., & Girolametto, L. (1992). Reassessing parent-focused language intervention programs. In S. Warren & J. Reichle (Eds.), *Causes and effects in communication and language intervention* (pp. 49-76). Baltimore: Brookes.

Warren, S., & Kaiser, A. (1986). Incidental language teaching: A critical review. *Journal of Speech and Hearing Disorders, 49*, 43-52.

Warren, S., F., Yoder, P. J., & Leew, S. V. (2002). Promoting social-communicative development in infants and toddlers. In H. Goldstein, L. A. Kaczmarek, & K. M. English (Eds.), *Communication and Language Intervention Series Volume 10, Promoting Social communication: Children with developmental disabilities from birth to adolescence.* Baltimore: Brookes.

Weiss, A. L. (1997) Planning language intervention for young children. In D. Bernstein & E. Tiegerman-Farber (Eds.), *Language and communication disorders in children* (4th Ed.). (pp.272-323). Boston: Allyn & Bacon.

Weiss, A. L. (2001). *Preschool language disorders resource guide: Specific language impairment.* San Diego: Singular.

CHAPTER 7

Focusing on Caregiver Participation in Intervention

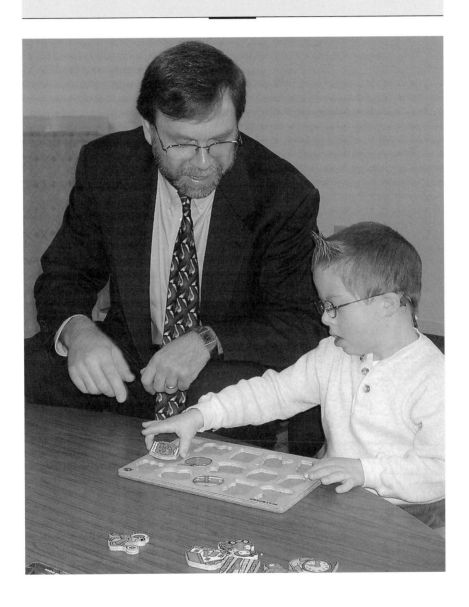

OUTLINE

PARENT-CAREGIVER AS SEEKER OF
  INFORMATION
PARENT-CAREGIVER AS LANGUAGE-
  INTERACTION FACILITATOR
  Parent-Caregiver's Responsiveness to
    Infant-Child Behavior and Facilitating
    the Interaction
  Parent-Caregiver's Use of Techniques to
    Facilitate Communication or Language

PARENT-CAREGIVER AS FACILITATOR OF
  PRELITERACY DEVELOPMENT
PARENT-CAREGIVER AS PARENT-
  CAREGIVER
CROSS-CULTURAL ISSUES IN PARENT-
  CAREGIVER INVOLVEMENT
SUMMARY

Parent and caregiver participation is considered the best practice in early intervention. This chapter presents information about different ways in which the family or caregiver can be involved in the intervention process. There are many models of family involvement in the intervention process. Parents have assumed many different roles in early intervention, depending on the model used for intervention and the degree to which the family desires to become involved in the intervention process. In accordance with the philosophy of this text, this chapter focuses on the major role that caregivers can assume in developing language and communication. Specifically, the chapter focuses on teaching the skills required to render an adult highly responsive to an infant or toddler's communicative attempts as well as the techniques to facilitate communication and language.

This chapter reviews the ways in which parents and caregivers become involved in early intervention. A key idea to keep in mind is that the amount of participation in early intervention is based on the involvement level the family wishes to assume. It should be noted that the long-term outcome of intervention is not contingent on the role that the parents and caregivers assume (Eiserman, Weber, & McCoun, 1995). The first way in which parents or caregivers can be involved in the early intervention process is to assume a role of seeker of information. Another model focuses on having the parent or caregiver become the facilitator of the interaction. Within these different models this chapter reviews various intervention techniques that have been used to encourage parents or caregivers to be actively involved in the intervention process.

PARENT-CAREGIVER AS SEEKER OF INFORMATION

The first way that parents and caregivers can be involved in early intervention is by assuming the role of seeker of information. This feeds nicely into the standard approach of parent involvement of parent education. Many interventionists feel comfortable with involving the family at this level, thus providing families with information about the child's handicapping condition, developmental expectations, and intervention techniques. Mahoney, Kaiser, Girolametto, MacDonald, Robinson, Safford & Spiker (1999) reported on research into the types of early intervention services that families want and found that "mothers' highest preferences were for parent education activities (child information and family instruction activities)" (p. 135). Best practices in early intervention would have us supplement parent education by providing the family with resources and information on issues that are concerns of the family relative to the child's needs and development.

Kaiser, Mahoney, Girolametto, MacDonald, Robinson, Safford & Spiker (1999) defined parent education as "the systematic provision of information to parents for the purpose of supporting their efforts to enhance their child's development" (p. 174). These authors further indicate that "parents from a range of socioeconomic backgrounds ... can and do seek information related to improving their effectiveness addressing the developmental and socio-emotional needs of their children" (p. 175). This view of parent education with the parent as seeker of information encompasses the view that parents will acquire information about their child's handicapping condition along with knowledge and skills that allow them to become involved in the intervention with their child. An important skill that the parent who is a seeker of information may need to develop is the ability to observe their infant or toddler. Being able to observe one's child is the first step in being able to identify and provide the information that the caregiver needs.

According to Mahoney et al. (1999), the primary goal of parent education is to instruct rather than to support the parent. Mahoney et al. also indicated that parent education is multifaceted in that the content of what is taught is diverse, which implies that the expected outcomes of parent education programs cover a range of options. Mahoney et al. indicated that the content encompasses a wide range of issues, from providing information about a child's current level of development and learning needs to instructing parents in the implementation of a variety of strategies to facilitate the child's functioning. The expected outcomes of parent education programs are equally diverse ranging from the expectation of increased parental knowledge to the child's acquisition of specific skills (p. 136). See Mahoney et al. for a more detailed discussion of the content and outcomes of various parent education programs.

Another purpose of parent education, as described by McCollum, Gooler, Appl, and Yates (2001), is "to enhance developmental opportunities for the child by expanding on and strengthening the parent–child relationship. This is accomplished by providing parents with information and support for being sensitive and responsive to their child's characteristics and development" (p. 37). This parent intervention program is based on the following general assumptions, which are then used as guides:

- Parent–child interaction is a critical context for early learning and development.
- The child, the parent, as well as the environment influence the parent–child interaction.
- Intervention can increase a parent's ability to read and respond to the infant's cues.
- The ability to read and respond to infant cues is contingent on knowledge and understanding of the infant's characteristics (McCollum et al., 2001)

This program incorporates the above assumptions by providing information on key topics associated with child development and then providing parents and caregivers opportunities to observe their child in relation to the topic presented in the parent session. Targeted observation is a key component of parent education programs.

Specifically, speech–language pathologists are interested in helping the parent or caregiver learn about basic communicative interactive patterns. It is crucial that caregivers know about prelinguistic communicative interactions as well as communicative interactions with the infant or child whose language is emerging. This information fits well into parent education programs about child development. Many programs include directed observation of the infant in either live or videotaped caregiver–infant interactions. Commercially available programs or videotapes can be used, but it is suggested that these materials be supplemented with direct instruction and discussion with the early interventionists. Direct contact with the speech–language pathologist should assure caregivers that they are not the cause of their infant's communicative difficulties, but rather that their infant may be very difficult to read and therefore difficult to interact with. The caregiver should not feel guilty and should know that he or she is not blamed. Positive encouragement and additional information can facilitate the process of having the parent develop positive communicative environments and interactions.

PARENT-CAREGIVER AS LANGUAGE-INTERACTION FACILITATOR

Another way in which parents and caregivers can be involved in the intervention process focuses on the role of the parent not as seeker of information but rather as receiver of information about how to strengthen the parent–child relationship or promote the parent–child interaction. Some have termed this type of parent education parent-mediated intervention (Mahoney et al., 1999). McCollum et al. (2001) indicated that the "parent–child interaction offers an especially powerful focus and context for early intervention by providing opportunities to define and support experiences that the two members of an interaction dyad have on one another and to work toward a strong relationship base for ongoing development" (p. 37).

Parent–child interaction intervention programs have focused on having the children experience responsive interactions. Girolametto, Weitzman, Wiigs, and Pearce (1999) have called these language programs the interactive model of language intervention. According to Warren (2000), there is increasing evidence that "suggests that highly responsive parenting styles foster the development of communication and language skills, as well as other important skills related to self-concept and emotional growth" (p. 34). Responsive interaction techniques have also been referred to as focused stimulation (Leonard, 1981) and interactive modeling (Wilcox, Kouri, & Cowell, 1991). These intervention programs have taught parents how to be responsive by employing a number of different techniques. A review of these techniques is presented later in this chapter.

As indicated earlier, the major role that caregivers can assume in developing language and communication is that of learning the skills needed to be highly responsive to an infant or toddler's communicative attempts as well as the techniques to facilitate communication and language.

Parent-Caregiver's Responsiveness to Infant-Child Behavior and Facilitating the Interaction

Parents and caregivers are responsive to behaviors that they consider communicative whether or not such behaviors are considered communicative by researchers (Yoder, Warren, McCathren, & Leew, 1998). There are intervention programs that focus on the responsiveness of parents and caregivers. The notion of having an intervention program focus on responsiveness and, in a larger sense, on having the parent or caregiver become the facilitator of the interaction is built on the notion that the expression of communicative intent is one of the building blocks of communicative expression and that communicative interaction can be both nonverbal (prelinguistic) and verbal (linguistic). Thus the focus of these intervention programs has been on developing the parent or caregiver's ability to facilitate the communicative interaction. These intervention models and programs can be divided into techniques and strategies that facilitate the infant or toddler's engagement in prelinguistic communicative interactions and those that can promote verbal (linguistic) interaction.

Facilitation of the infant or toddler's engagement in prelinguistic communicative interactions is built on the premise that caregivers need to respond to the infant or toddler's communicative intent or act and that caregivers should be contingently responsive to the infant from birth. The first step in so doing requires that the parent or caregiver recognize the infant's physiological state and readiness to communicate. Rossetti (1990) indicated that the infant's state could be defined as the "level of alertness and environmental interaction patterns present in an infant or toddler at any given point" (p. 106). Brazelton and Nugent (1995) indicated that there are six infant states. These are: (1) deep or quiet sleep, (2) light or active sleep, (3) drowsy, semidozing, (4) quiet alert, (5) active awake, and (6) crying.

Gorski, Davison, and Brazelton (1979) indicated that the infant's state determines whether the infant is ready to participate in interaction. The infant should be at least in stage 4 to respond to environmental stimuli or interaction. Parents and caregivers can determine their infant's state through observation and use the quiet alert stage as an opportunity to begin communicative interactions. It is during the quiet alert stage that the parent or caregiver may be better able to engage the baby's attention and elicit reciprocity (Paul, 2001).

Parents need to develop skills that will help them interpret their infant's communicative behavior. Parents tend to interact more with infants who smile and vocalize at them. If a parent is unresponsive to his or her infant, that individual might need help to become aware of the infant's readable communicative signals. Dunst and Lowe (1986) indicated that readability is the extent to which an infant produces distinctive behaviors and that readability determines the extent to which caregivers can respond to these behaviors as communicative. We know that an infant's behaviors are readable when parents and caregivers can confidently say, "Oh, he's tired." The extent to which the caregiver can read the infant's signals leads to the caregiver's feelings of effectiveness. It takes the parent or caregiver longer to decide how to respond to the infant who is difficult to read, and this may result in less contingent interactions between parent or caregiver and infant. Dunst and Lowe (1986) indicated that caregivers can develop the skills to help them "read" their infant's behavior. A caregiver who reads the infant's behavior as intents to communicate will respond to the child in a contingent manner. Yoder et al. (1998) indicated that there are three types of parent or caregiver responsiveness: nonlinguistic contingent responses, linguistic contingent responses to the child's focus of attention, and linguistic contingent responses to the child's communicative act (p. 40).

Dunst and Lowe (1986) suggested that interactive coaching enhances a caregiver's ability to engage in effective, well-balanced interactions with their infant. Interactive teaching includes instructing parents on how to read the behavior of their infant as communicative and then to respond contingently. Specific techniques include having the caregiver initiate an interaction, wait, respond contingently, and imitate the infant's behavior as a means of establishing a reciprocal pattern of interaction. As indicated above, these contingent responses can be linguistic or nonlinguistic. Yoder et al. (1998) reported that "babies of mothers who used relatively high levels of non-linguistic responding tend to be highly social, securely attached, loquacious, and less distressed" (p. 45) and that nonlinguistic maternal responding facilitates an infant's learning. Yoder et al. (1998) also reported that caregivers who responded linguistically to their infants' focus of attention (usually by labeling) facilitated the child's acquisition of nouns.

Dunst and Lowe (1986) suggested three techniques that can be introduced to the parent or caregiver to put infant and caregiver in touch with one another: (1) increase readability, (2) recognize the infant or toddler's reasons for communicating, and (3) respond to readable and predictable cues. To increase readability it is suggested that the child be placed in situations that provide the infant with experiences requiring communicative behavior as part of the event or activity and making continuation of the event or activity possible. If the readability of the infant is low, the caregiver should repeat and consistently respond to the infant's behavior as if it is communicative. Landry, Smith, Miller-Loncar, and Swank (1998) indicated that caregivers should "provide specialized assistance ('scaffolding') by controlling the learning task so infants can attend to components within their range of capability" (p. 105). Thus the parent or caregiver can gradually require more conventional communicative behavior; most important is that the infant experiences activities or events that have communicative behavior as a critical part of the event or activity, and that the caregiver or parents' responses are invariable. A similar technique suggested by Yoder and Warren (1993) is for adults to respond contingently to the child's current communication behaviors about an activity or event in which the child shows interest. Yoder and Warren indicated that this responsiveness to prelinguistic behavior is facilitative of communication development because it enhances the infant or toddler's communicative effectiveness and productiveness by developing the child's understanding that communication affects the behavior of others.

Paul (2001) indicates that there are four types of interactive behaviors that caregivers of prelinguistic infants should develop. These include turn taking, imitation, establishing joint attention, and developing anticipatory sets.

To be able to take turns with his or her infant, the caregiver must recognize the infant's communicative signals or readiness to interact. Turn taking can consist of the caregiver's vocalizing and smiling at the infant and waiting for the infant to respond. If the infant responds in any manner, the caregiver should imitate the response. The infant's behavior need not be a smile or a vocalization; it can be a head movement. The caregiver's response should be an imitation of the infant's behavior. For more information about establishing turn taking and responding to any infant behavior, see MacDonald's Ecological Communication (ECO) program (Gillette & MacDonald, 1989; MacDonald & Gillette, 1989).

Yoder and Warren (1993) also suggested that parents and caregivers engage in contingent imitation as a first step toward developing their child's communication. According to Yoder and Warren (1993), the benefits to the child are that "it allows him or her to regulate the amount of social stimulation received, increases the probability that adult input will be easily processed and understood, and may encourage the child to imitate the adult's behavior" (p. 44). These authors also suggested that the result of engaging in contingent imitation may be the child's greater attention to the social partner, increased vocal and verbal imitation, and increased exploratory play, including more differentiated play schemes.

Establishing joint focus of attention is another important skill that parents and caregivers should develop (Paul, 2001). Joint focus of attention suggests that the caregiver and child are focusing on the same object or event at the same time. Bruner (1981) first emphasized the importance of establishing joint attention as a means of sharing the topic of the conversation or interaction. In typical child-centered interactions, once joint attention is established, parents or caregivers tend to label the item of focus or make a comment about the item of focus, thus establishing the topic of the interaction (conversation). Owens (2001) indicated that joint attention can exist in two formats: indicating or marking. In *indicating,* the parent follows the infant's line of regard or visual attention and then comments on the object of their joint attention. With *marking,* the parent shakes an object or exaggerates an action to attract the infant's attention and then labels or comments on the shared focus of attention.

The establishment of anticipatory sets provides the infant with a predictable series of sound and action, which in turn provide a structure within which the infant can analyze language. Early examples of joint action can be found in the anticipatory games, such as peek-a-boo, that caregivers play with their infants. It should be noted that these infant games are culturally determined, and the speech–language pathologist needs to determine which infant games are part of the caregiver's culture.

Another part of this notion of reading the child's communicative intent and placing the child in a supportive and encouraging communicative interaction is the nature of the interaction itself. Leonard (1992) recommended that increasing successful communicative interactions may be accomplished by altering the adult's responsiveness to the child's communication attempts or by establishing routines in which the child can successfully participate. Yoder and Warren (1993) also suggested using social routines as an intervention context. Routines are predictable and include turn-taking games and rituals such as "peek-a-boo" or "pat-a-cake." Warren and Yoder (1998) indicated that social routines can be built through arranging the environment and following the child's lead. The environment should be arranged to increase the probability that the infant or toddler will engage in communicative behavior, either to initiate communicative interactions or to respond to a parent or caregiver's initiation (Donahue-Kilburg, 1992). Routines can be established as part of daily activities or can be unique to a particular child. The predictable structure of the routine may help the infant or toddler remember the appropriate interactive role. Yoder and Warren (1993) indicated that "once the child learns the predictable role in a routine, he or she can devote greater attention to analyzing adult models of new ways to communicate" (p. 45). In addition, the salience of "adult models may be enhanced because slight variations in the routine create a moderately novel situation that is particularly salient to the child" (p. 45).

When working with parents or caregivers to facilitate verbal communicative interaction, a number of components of verbal communication must be considered. Wilcox and Shannon (1998) suggested that "specific communication behavior targets must be identified to facilitate parental models and responses" (p. 403). The strategies that can be used by parents or caregivers depend somewhat on the specific targeted behavior. Wilcox and Shannon (1998) indicated that the strategies taught to parents can be milieu techniques or responsive interaction techniques.

Kaiser, Hemmeter, Ostrosky, Fischer, Yoder & Keefer (1996), in a program where parents were taught to implement responsive interaction techniques, found that all of the children in their study increased the use of targeted language structures. The study also found that the caregivers maintained the use of the facilitation strategies 6 months after the intervention program and that the increases in the children's language were also maintained. An additional important aspect of this study was that the parents included in the study reported high levels of satisfaction in the intervention outcomes and with their participation in the training experiences.

In summary, the skills needed for parents or caregivers to read their infant's behavior as communicative include the following:

- Parents and caregivers should recognize the infant or toddler's physiological state and readiness to communicate.
- Parents and caregivers should recognize the infant or toddler's behaviors as intents to communicate.
- Parents and caregivers should respond to the infant or toddler's cues that have communicative potential nonlinguistically and linguistically.
- Techniques needed by parents and caregivers to put them in touch with their infant or toddler are to increase readability, recognize the child's reasons for communicating, and respond to readable and predictable cues.

- Parents and caregivers should use social routines as the intervention context.

Parent-Caregiver's Use of Techniques to Facilitate Communication or Language

Tannock and Girolametto (1992) reviewed the literature on parent-focused language intervention and presented a delineation of three types of intervention techniques that can be used by the parent or caregiver to facilitate their child's language development. The three types of intervention techniques are child-oriented techniques, interaction-promoting techniques, and language-modeling techniques. The combination of these three types of techniques is believed to foster the child's development of early communicative, socio-interactional, and linguistic skills. In the child-oriented techniques the parent or caregiver focuses on the child's interest, object of attention, or interactional or conversational topic. By being child oriented, these techniques fine-tune the complexity of the caregiver's input to the child's level of functioning. The interaction-promoting techniques focus on the turn-taking nature of the interaction so that the child experiences the roles of both interaction initiator and maintainer. A key component of the interaction-promoting techniques is the establishment of balanced turn taking between the child and the parent or caregiver. The language-modeling techniques used by the parent or caregiver provide the infant or toddler with the linguistic means to express the relations between form, content, and use. Specifically, these language-modeling techniques provide the child with simple linguistic input that is presented at the moment the child experiences an environmental action, an interest, or a focus of attention, and is meaningfully related to that action, interest, or focus of attention.

Another model for incorporating parents into early intervention is joint book reading. Dale, Crain-Thoreson, Notari-Syverson, and Cole (1996) indicated that parents provide more complex and sophisticated language during story time, emphasize the informational function of language, and engage in vocabulary teaching. The context of book reading provides the caregiver with a known context, so that it is easier for the caregiver to respond contingently. The specific techniques that were presented to parents to facilitate language include the following:

- Ask *what* questions.
- Follow the child's answer with questions.
- Repeat what the child says.
- Ask open-ended questions.
- Expand on what the child says.
- Help the child as needed.
- Praise and encourage the child.
- Shadow the child's interests.
- Have fun (Dale et al., 1996, based on Whitehurst et al., 1988).

In this program is a repetition of the notion of following the child's lead, ("shadow the child's interests") as well as the techniques of imitation ("repeat what the child says" and "expand on what the child says"). However, more specific directive techniques are taught to parents. These include asking *what* questions, as well as open-ended questions, and following a child's response with a question.

McNeil and Fowler (1999) implemented a program that taught caregivers to use praise, expansions, open-ended questions, and pauses for initiation during book reading. Caregivers used the strategies that were highlighted in this program; use of these strategies resulted in increases in the number of conversations the children engaged in during book reading, as well as in the number of child turns during the conversation. Once again the strategy of expansion, whether during play or book reading, seems to facilitate children's use of language. However, in both of these studies the benefit of using more directive techniques is evident (e.g., asking *what* or open-ended questions).

Use of these more directive techniques is discouraged in the interactive model described previously. The use of directives, though not encouraged in the interactive language intervention model, has been found to be a strategy used by caregivers when interacting with more passive and inactive children (Girolametto, 1995). Girolametto (1995) reported that some parents use directiveness as an "adaptive strategy to promote joint action, attention and interaction" (p. 104).

Kaiser (1993) suggested a hybrid model for parent-implemented intervention programs. The model incorporates information on milieu teaching (a more directive model), environmental support for language learning, and information on responsive and interactive models. The model has three components: environmental arrangement, responsive interaction strategies, and milieu teaching strategies. The environmental arrangement of this model is "designed to increase the child's engagement with the physical setting and with the parent or caregiver and to provide frequent opportunities for the parent or caregiver to communicate with the child" (p. 75). The parent or caregiver is taught how to select toys and materials of high interest to the child and to join the child in play. Once the caregiver is engaged with the child, the intervention program moves to the second component of responsive interaction instruction. Parents and caregivers learn "basic principles of inter-action (responsiveness, following the child's lead, facilitating turn taking, matching and extending the child's topic) and basic language modeling strategies (matching the child's linguistic level, imitating or mirroring the child, expansions of the child's utterances, descriptive talk)" (p. 76). The final component of this model is teaching the milieu strategies. The milieu strategies are language facilitator controlled and thus are a more direct language-teaching approach.

Two specific parent intervention programs that are well documented in the literature are the Hanen program (Manolson, 1992) and the ECO program developed by MacDonald and Gillette (1989).

The Hanen program stresses parental participation in intervention. Under-lying the program is the belief that parents are the best language facilitators because parents spend the most time with their children, know their children the best, and have emotional commitment to their children. The main purposes of the program are to educate parents about language development and how to teach their children who have language delays how to commu-nicate, to help parents develop the skills needed to facilitate their child's language and communication development, and to provide support to parents (by providing the information to parents in group sessions). The specific language facilitation techniques that this program promotes include allowing the child to lead, adapting to the child's focus of attention or sharing the moment, and adding information to the child's communication attempt.

- To follow the child's lead, the parents will observe the child's focus of attention, waiting for the child to express himself or herself, and listen carefully to the child's attempts to communicate.
- To share the moment, parents are encouraged to be face to face with their child, to use strategies that let their child know they are listening (by imitating the child, interpreting the child's communication, and making comments), and to encourage turn taking or a conversational format.
- To add information to the conversation, parents are encouraged to respond to the child by using imitation, labeling, expansion, commenting, clarification, and repetition.

The *Ecological Program for Communication* (Gillette & MacDonald, 1989; MacDonald & Gillette, 1989) is designed as a partnership program between parents (caregivers) and intervention personnel (speech–language pathologists). The principles underlying the program "address how adults interact and communicate with children so that the children learn to be social and communicative with them" (MacDonald, 1989, p. 20). As part of the program the adult should develop a balanced give-and-take relationship or partnership with the child, match the child's developmental communicative level, respond to the child's communication, and be nondirective when interacting with the child. Gillette (1989) described the four steps in the intervention process. Step one involves assessment of the parent–child play–communication partnership through observation and interview. Step two involves the development of an intervention plan to develop the parent–child partnership as well as to educate the parent or caregiver as to the reasons underlying the principles of the program (e.g., educate the parent on the impact of his or her behavior on the child's communication). Step three involves practice. It should be noted that step three suggests a specific mode of parent training. Gillette (1989) suggested that the interventionist demonstrate an activity (or a specific strategy) for the parent and observe the parent doing the same activity (strategy) with the child. The interventionist should then give the parent feedback that is brief and focuses first on positive aspects of the observation prior to giving comments on related problems. The final step involves integrating the treatment into daily life. The goal of the fourth step is to bridge the gap between the clinic and the natural learning environment so that the parent or caregiver will use what has been learned in this program to interact and communicate with their child on a routine basis.

A more specific eclectic model is suggested here that incorporates the tenets of Tannock and Girolametto (1992), as well as those of Dale et al. (1996), MacDonald (1985), MacDonald and Gillette (1989), and Manolson (1992). This modified interaction-focused intervention program takes into account the literature that focuses on the parent or caregiver responding to the infant or toddler's communicative intent or act (e.g., being contingently responsive to the infant [from the first day]). To do this, the parent or caregiver must observe the infant or toddler to determine the child's focus of attention, interest, or potential conversational topic. The parent is striving for joint attention at this time. Once the parent or caregiver can identify the child's focus of attention, interest, or conversational topic, he or she should respond to the infant in ways that facilitate the interaction. At this point, use of the interaction-promoting techniques of Tannock and Girolametto (1992) is suggested, and the parent or caregiver also should assign communicative intent to the infant or toddler's behavior and format the interaction into a conversation. To do so, the parent or caregiver must respond to the child. These responses should be within the child's "proximal zone of development" (the parent should respond at the outer limits of the child's stage of development but not too far above it). The responses include the following:

- Acknowledgment or affirmation: The parent or caregiver should let the infant know that his or her focus of attention is being recognized and accepted.
- Nonverbal response: A nonverbal response can be a touch, a look, a smile, anything that lets the infant know that the adult is responding in a positive manner.
- Translate the child's unconventional acts.
- Repeat what the child says.
- Expand what the child says.
- Extend what the child says.
- Signal turn exchange.

Refer to Table 7-1 for a more detailed list of the interactive techniques that can be employed by caregivers.

Another aspect of this model, focusing on the interaction, requires that the parent or caregiver provide the infant or toddler with the form to encode his or her communicative intent. When parents and caregivers provide the form of the message they are using language-modeling techniques, and these techniques are described in the literature (Owens, 1999; Weiss, 2001). A final aspect of this model requires the caregivers to think about environmental arrangements to provide the physical context in which they can engage with their child in play and facilitate language and communication.

When the parent or caregiver of a very young infant does not think there is communicative intent, or if the intent of the message is unclear and ambiguous, the parent or caregiver should assign intent to the child. In addition, the parent or caregiver also should translate the child's unconventional act into a meaningful, standardized communicative act. There are two ways that the parent or caregiver can do this: (1) repeat what the child has done, and (2) model the message. If the infant or child is expressing something, the parent or caregiver's role changes to repeating, expanding, or extending the child's communicative message. The simplest way in which the parent can provide the form of the message is to repeat what the child has said, using a standard model. To expand the child's communicative message means to rephrase it, and to extend the child's communicative message is to add information that is relevant to the joint focus of attention or the presumed conversational topic. This interaction extension of the parent-training model merges with the second role parents and caregivers can assume.

Another aspect of the parent or caregiver's role in intervention should focus on the adult's interaction style. Adults should have a variety of interaction styles so that the child is exposed to multiple ways in which language can be

Table 7-1	*Interactive techniques*
TYPE OF TECHNIQUE	**EXAMPLES**
Child-Oriented Techniques	– respond to the child's focus of attention – follow the child's lead – match child's style and abilities – enter child's world by situating self at same physical level, maintain face to face interaction, establish eye contact, playing, being animated
Interaction-Promoting Techniques	– take one turn at a time – wait with anticipation – signal for turns – decrease directiveness – imitate the child's turn (to keep the interaction moving) – model – turnabout – balance the communicative turns – match
Language Modeling Techniques	– comment on activities of child and self – use contingent labeling – use short, simple utterances – use repetition – expand or extend the child's turn – buildup and breakdown – recast

Adapted from Tannock, R. & Girolametto, L. (1992). Reassessing parent-focused language intervention programs. In S. Warren & J. Reichle (Eds.), *Causes and effects in Communication and language intervention*. Baltimore: Brooks.

used to communicate. The focus of the intervention described thus far has been on responsiveness and fun during the interaction. Yet as the infant begins to use language, he or she should be exposed to the use of language to inform, to explain, to express feelings and intent, to pretend and imagine, and to talk about the future (Weitzman, 1992).

PARENT-CAREGIVER AS FACILITATOR OF PRELITERACY DEVELOPMENT

Previously, the context of joint book reading was discussed as an appropriate context in which caregivers can facilitate language. This context is appropriate for enhancing the language of typical children, as well as for enhancing that of children with delayed language (McNeill & Fowler, 1999). However, another important aspect of joint book reading is that it also can be a context in which the caregiver fosters preliteracy skills. During joint book reading, caregivers "engage in a variety of cognitive and linguistic behaviors intended to encourage their child's participation in the act of reading" (Martin & Reutzel, 1999, p. 39). Young children develop many skills during preliteracy activities (book sharing when the child is in the early stages of developing language). Some of the skills include phonological awareness, letter knowledge, word awareness (vocabulary development), book conventions, narrative development, and, eventually, abstract language development. With prelinguistic children the majority of the caregiver's behavior is focused on getting and maintaining the child's attention. Martin and Reutzel (1999) found that mothers shared control of the text, such as holding the book or turning the pages, to maintain the child's attention to the book-reading activity. In addition, Martin and Reutzel indicated that mothers spent more time in attention getting and maintaining behaviors with the younger children; however, use of these behaviors began to decrease by the time the children reached 24 months. Mothers also used other strategies when engaging in joint book reading to encourage the child's participation. Included in these strategies were text simplifications and elaborations. Reasons for a mother's simplifying the text included simplification of the language, the mother's perceptions about the child's past experience, and modifications in the mother's reading of the text (Martin & Reutzel, 1999). Reasons for a mother's elaborating on the book text included teaching new concepts, relating new concepts to past experiences, problem solving, reviewing concepts, and reinforcing concepts (Martin & Reutzel, 1999).

PARENT-CAREGIVER AS PARENT-CAREGIVER

A final suggestion is that parents and caregivers be encouraged to enjoy the child without all of the baggage that is sometimes associated with having a child with special needs. Leonard (1992) suggested that early interventionists should remember to increase the number of enjoyable and successful communications between the child and family members. The result of successful communication will be reduced frustration on the part of both the child and the family. Successful interaction between the family and the child may also result in a stronger bond between parent and child.

CROSS-CULTURAL ISSUES IN PARENT-CAREGIVER INVOLVEMENT

When the early interventionist works with parents and caregivers and provides the family with information about strengthening or facilitating the parent– or caregiver–child interaction, it should be remembered that family values, beliefs, and interaction styles vary based on cultural expectations. Not all families are willing to initiate the intervention process or become involved in the intervention itself, and some families may have concerns. Hammer and Weiss (2000) indicated that "providing suggestions to parents about how to interact with their children has implications for parents that go beyond the immediate setting and may run counter to their cultural beliefs about their children's language development" (p. 127). The interventionist can overcome a family's sense that being provided with interaction information may run counter to their culture by carefully reviewing information about their values, beliefs, desires, and interaction styles before beginning this course of intervention. Ellis Weismer (2000) indicated that interventionists should develop "an appreciation of the sociolinguistic or pragmatic rules concerning the makeup of social interaction" (p.185) when working with families from culturally or linguistically diverse backgrounds. Warren, Yoder, and Leew (2002) suggested that the interventionist review all families' values, beliefs, and desires regardless of cultural and ethnic background. Anderson and Battle (1998) took this view a step further by indicating that each family "must be regarded as a cultural unit with its own values, beliefs, and practices, which may be shared with the larger cultural group or may be unique to the family" (pp. 214-215). Hammer and Weiss (2000) suggested the use of ethnographic or semistructured interviews, as well as observation, as a means of obtaining the information about each family's values, beliefs, and practices. Thus the interventionist must be cognizant of each family's individual cultural and ethnic background and ask each family about their cultural values, beliefs, and practices that are relevant to the communicative development of their child. The interventionist can then tailor the intervention program to the individual family and by so doing provide culturally competent services.

SUMMARY

This chapter describes some of the roles that parents and caregivers can assume during the intervention process. These roles have focused on the parent and caregiver's participation in the intervention. However, other researchers have described additional roles that parents or caregivers can take that include the following: parent or caregiver as observer, parent or caregiver as parent or caregiver facilitator, and parent or caregiver as advocate (Tiegerman-Farber, 1995). When the parent or caregiver is an observer, he or she becomes a critical reporter of information; this role was elaborated on earlier in this text. Parents or caregivers as parent facilitators are an important part of the intervention process because they can share information with others who have had similar experiences. Parents or caregivers can also become advocates, and they can understand the importance of their involvement in their child's life and take an active role throughout it.

It should be noted that not all families want to be involved in the intervention process, and some may even be hostile to the efforts of the early interventionist. McWilliam (1996) indicated that these families "would prefer that we not be involved in their lives, but have been coerced by another agency into receiving our services" (p. 146). In these cases the interventionist should work on developing trust and hope that eventually the family will be involved in some aspects of the intervention process.

REFERENCES

Anderson, N., & Battle, D. E. (1998). Culturally diverse families and the development of language. In D. E. Battle (Ed.), *Communication disorders in multicultural populations* (2nd Ed.) (pp. 213-246). Boston: Butterworth-Heinemann.

Brazelton, T. B., & Nugent, J. K. (1995). *Neonatal behavioral assessment scale* (3rd Ed). Cambridge, MA: Cambridge University Press.

Bruner, J. (1981). The social context of language acquisition. *Language and Communication, 1*, 155-178.

Dale, P. S., Crain-Thoreson, C., Notari-Syverson, A., & Cole, K. (1996). Parent–child book reading as an intervention technique for young children with language delays. *Topics in Early Childhood Special Education, 16*(2), 213-235.

Donahue-Kilburg (1992). *Family-centered early intervention for communication disorders: Prevention and treatment.* Gaithersburg, MD: Aspen.

Dunst, C. J., & Lowe, L. W. (1986). From reflex to symbol: Describing, explaining and fostering communicative competence. *AAC Augmentative and Alternative Communication, 2*(1), 11-18.

Eiserman, W. D., Weber, C., & McCoun, M. (1995). Parent and professional roles in early intervention: A longitudinal comparison of the effects of two intervention configurations. *Journal of Special Education, 29*(1), 20-44.

Ellis Weismer, S. (2000). Language intervention for young children with language impairments. In L. R. Watson, E. Crais, & T. L. Layton (Eds.), *Handbook of early language impairment in children: Assessment and treatment* (pp. 173-198). Albany, NY: Delmar Thomson Learning.

Gillette, Y. (1989). *Ecological programs for communicating partnerships: Models and cases.* San Antonio, TX: Special Press.

Gillette, Y., & MacDonald, J. (1989). *ECO resources: Using the ECO model for communicating partnerships.* Itasca, IL: Riverside.

Girolametto, L. (1995). Reflection on the origins of directiveness: Implications for intervention. *Journal of Early Intervention, 19*(2), 104-106.

Girolametto, L., Weitzman, E., Wiigs, M., & Pearce, P. S. (1999). The relationship between maternal language measures and language development in toddlers with expressive language delays. *American Journal of Speech–Language Pathology, 8*(4), 364-374.

Gorski, P., Davison, M., & Brazelton, B. (1979). Stages of behavioral organization in the high risk neonate: Theoretical and clinical considerations. *Seminars in Perinatology, 3*, 61.

Hammer, C. S., & Weiss, A. L. (2000). African American mothers' views of their infants' language development and language-learning environment. *American Journal of Speech–Language Pathology, 9*(2), 126-140.

Kaiser, A. P. (1993). Parent-implemented language intervention: An environmental system perspective. In A. P. Kaiser & D. B. Bray (Eds.) *Enhancing children's communication: Research foundations for intervention* (pp. 63-84). Baltimore: Brookes.

Kaiser, A. P., Hemmeter, M. L., Ostrosky, M. M., Fischer, R., Yoder, P., & Keefer, M. (1996). The effects of teaching parents to use responsive interaction strategies. *Topics in Early Childhood Special Education, 16*(3), 375-406.

Kaiser, A.P., Mahoney, G., Girolametto, L., MacDonald, J., Robinson, C., Safford, D., & Spiker, D. (1999). Rejoinder: Toward a contemporary vision of parent education. *Topics in Early Childhood Special Education, 19*(3), 173-176.

Landry, S. H., Smith, K. E., Miller-Loncar, C. L., & Swank, P. R. (1998). The relation of change in maternal interactive styles to the developing social competence of full-term and preterm children. *Child Development, 69*(1), 105-123.

Leonard, L. (1981). Facilitating linguistic skills in children with specific language impairment. *Applied Linguistics, 2*, 89-118.

Leonard, J. S. (1992). Communication intervention for young children at risk for specific communication disorders. *Seminars in Speech and Language, 13*(3), 223-236.

MacDonald, J. (1989). *Becoming partners with children: From play to conversation.* San Antonio, TX: Special Press.

MacDonald, J. (1985). Language through conversation: A model for intervention with language-delayed persons. In S. Warren & A. Roger-Warren (Eds.), *Teaching functional language* (pp. 89-122). Baltimore: University Park Press.

MacDonald, J., & Gillette, Y. (1989). *An introduction to the Ecological Communication Program*. Itasca, IL: Riverside.

Mahoney, G., Kaiser, A., Girolametto, L., MacDonald, J., Robinson, C., Safford, P., & Spiker, D. (1999). Parent education in early intervention: A call for a renewed focus. *Topics in Early Childhood Special Education, 19*(3), 131-140.

Manolson, A. (1992). *It takes two to talk*. Bisbee, AZ: Imaginart.

Martin, L.E., & Reutzel, D.R. (1999). Sharing books: Examining how and why mothers deviate from the print. *Reading Research and Instruction, 39*(1), 39-70.

McCollum, J. A., Gooler, F., Appl, D. J., & Yates, T. J. (2001). PIWI: Enhancing parent–child interaction as a foundation for early intervention. *Infants and Young Children, 14*(1), 34-45.

McNeill, J. H. & Fowler, S. A. (1999). Let's talk: Encouraging mother-child conversations during story reading. *Journal of Early Intervention, 22*(1), 51-69.

McWilliam, P. J. (1996). Day-to-day service provision. In P. J. McWilliam, P. J. Winton, & E. R. Crais (Eds.), *Practical strategies for family-centered intervention* (pp. 125-154). San Diego: Singular.

Owens, R. (1999). *Language disorders: A functional approach to assessment and intervention* (3rd Ed). Boston: Allyn & Bacon.

Owens, R. (2001). *Language development: An introduction* (5th Ed). Boston: Allyn & Bacon.

Paul, R. (2001). *Language disorders from infancy through adolescence: Assessment and intervention* (2nd Ed). St Louis, MO: Mosby.

Rossetti, L. (1990). *Infant–toddler assessment: An interdisciplinary approach*. Boston: College Hill Press.

Tannock, R., & Girolametto, L. (1992). Reassessing parent-focused language intervention programs. In S. Warren & J. Reichle (Eds.), *Causes and effects in communication and language intervention* (pp. 49-76). Baltimore: Brookes.

Tiegerman-Farber, E. (1995). *Language and communication intervention in preschool children*. Boston: Allyn & Bacon.

Warren, S. F. (2000). The future of early communication and language intervention. *Topics in Early Childhood Special Education, 20*(1), 33-37.

Warren, S. F., & Yoder, P. J. (1998). Facilitating the transition from preintentional to intentional communication. In A. M. Wetherby, S. F. Warren, & J. Reichle (Eds.), *Transitions in prelinguistic communication* (pp.365-384). Baltimore: Brookes.

Warren, S. F., Yoder, P. J., & Leew, S. V. (2002). Promoting social-communicative development in infants and toddlers. In H. Goldstein, L. Kaczmarek, & K. English (Eds.), *Promoting social communication: Children with developmental disabilities from birth to adolescence* (pp. 121-150). Baltimore: Brookes.

Weiss, A. L. (2001). *Preschool Language disorders resource guide: Specific language impairment*. San Diego: Singular.

Weitzman E. (1992). *Learning language and loving it: A guide to promoting children's social and language development in early childhood settings*. Toronto: Hanen Center.

Wilcox, M. J., Kouri, T., & Caswell, S. (1991). Early language intervention: A comparison of classroom and individual treatment. *American Journal of Speech–Language Pathology, 1*, 49-62.

Wilcox, M. J. & Shannon, M. S. (1998). Facilitating the transition from prelinguistic to linguistic communication. In A. M. Wetherby, S. F. Warren, & J. Reichle (Eds.), *Transitions in prelinguistic communication* (pp. 385-416). Baltimore, MD: Paul H. Brookes Publishing Co.

Yoder, P. J., & Warren, S. F. (1993). Can developmentally delayed children's language development be enhanced through prelinguistic intervention? In A. P. Kaiser & D. B. Gray (Eds.), *Enhancing children's communication: Research foundations for intervention* (pp.35-61). Baltimore: Brookes.

Yoder, P. J., Warren, S. F., McCathren, R., & Leew, S. V. (1998). Does adult responsivity to child behavior facilitate communication development? In A.M. Wetherby, S. F. Warren, & J. Rechle (Eds.), *Transition in prelinguistic communication* (pp. 39-58). Baltimore: Brookes.

CHAPTER 8

Case Studies to Illustrate the Intervention Process

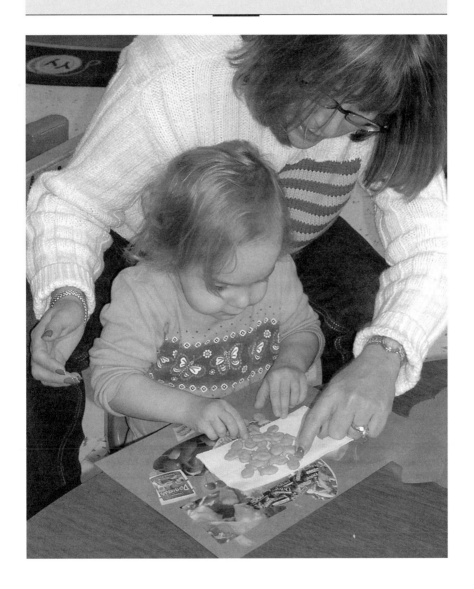

OUTLINE

INTERVENTION PLAN FOR JOSHUA P.	INTERVENTION PLAN FOR BRANDON Z.
Communication Outcome 1	Communication Outcome 1
Justification	Justification
Short-Term Objective Justification	Short-Term Objective Justification
Strategy: Caregiver as Language	Strategy: Phonological Skills
Facilitator	Communication Outcome 2
Communication Outcome 2	Justification
Justification	Short-Term Objective Justification
Short-Term Objective Justification	Strategy: Form of Expressing
Strategy: Communication Form	Communicative Intent
Communication Outcome 3	Communication Outcome 3
Justification	Justification
Short-Term Objective Justification	Short-Term Objective Justification
Strategy: Language Comprehension	Strategy: Receptive Language
and Symbolic Play	

This chapter discusses communication outcomes and short-term communication objectives, as well as the rationale for the communication outcomes and objectives. In addition, possible intervention strategies are presented, including both the event or activity in which intervention can take place and the language facilitation techniques that can be implemented. The purpose of this chapter is to translate the framework discussed in Chapters 5 through 7 to practical clinical practice.

INTERVENTION PLAN FOR JOSHUA P.

Communication Outcome 1

> Communication Outcome 1: Mrs. P. will learn language facilitation strategies and use them during daily activities.

Justification During play a positive interaction was noted between Mrs. P. and J.P. Mrs. P. commented on J.P.'s actions and vocalizations in relation to the context; thus, she appropriately labeled objects with which J.P. was playing. However, it was noted that little use was made of expansion or extension after the labeling of objects in the play context. During an interview on the subject of her interactions with J.P., Mrs. P. expressed feelings of frustration, such as when she labeled objects with which J.P. was playing and he did not say the word. Mrs. P. reported that she was finding herself demanding words from J.P., which resulted in J.P.'s playing independently rather than with her. This communication outcome focused on Mrs. P.'s learning to use strategies that would facilitate J.P.'s language development, since Mrs. P. had indicated her desire to be an effective partner in J.P.'s intervention program. This communication outcome was critical, since J.P. is being seen by the speech–language pathologist twice a week, whereas the rest of the time he is with his family, participating in the many daily activities that make up their lives. To provide J.P. with many opportunities to learn language, the involvement of the family is vital.

> **Short-Term Objective 1.1:** Mrs. P. will learn to imitate J.P.'s vocalizations and then expand them to simple words.
>
> **Short-Term Objective 1.2:** Mrs. P. will learn to follow J.P.'s lead during a play session and provide him with clear, simple, and specific information about the objects that are his focus of attention. She will use parallel talk to provide him with more than just the labels for the objects; thus she will also interpret his actions and gestures and expand and extend his expressive communication.

Short-Term Objective Justification As noted in Chapter 7, a caregiver's actions are critical to the child's language learning. The focus of these objectives is to develop Mrs. P.'s ability as a language facilitator. The specific techniques are tied to J.P.'s other communication outcomes; first, to Mrs. P.'s role in facilitating J.P.'s sound development and, second, to the development of J.P.'s linguistic knowledge.

Strategy: Caregiver as Language Facilitator Mrs. P. will have a hands-on approach similar to the Hanen method. Mrs. P. will be given written and verbal information about specific language facilitation techniques: following child's lead, imitating child's utterances, and modeling techniques (both expansion and extension). She will also be given videotapes that illustrate the use of the language facilitation techniques. A videotape of Mrs P.'s interaction with J.P. will then be made. The speech–language pathologist and caregiver will view the videotape separately and then together to identify the times Mrs. P. used one of the facilitation techniques, as well as additional opportunities in which she could employ one of the facilitation techniques. In collaboration the caregiver and speech–language pathologist will identify one daily event in which Mrs. P. may feel comfortable using one or more of the techniques.

Mrs. P. will also be encouraged to use self-talk and parallel talk to provide J.P. with focused stimulation to facilitate his language abilities.

Communication Outcome 2

> **Communication Outcome 2:** J.P. will increase the range and frequency of the form of his expressive communication.

Justification The primary reason to work on the form of J.P.'s communication is that at 15 months a child is expected to produce his or her first meaningful word. J.P. communicated primarily through gestures and very limited vocalizations. "Pointing and grunting are not as informative as words, children with expressive language delay experience much communication frustrations" (Whitehurst, Fischel, Arnold, & Lonigan, 1992, p. 297); therefore the form of J.P.'s communicative attempts should be developed. Specifically, J.P.'s progression toward the use of the conventional system of spoken communication should be encouraged. In addition, J.P.'s phonological skills should be developed to increase his production of consonant sounds, in accordance with Paul's (2001) assertion that expanding the consonant repertoire of children who are not yet using words will facilitate speech production.

> **Short-Term Objective 2.1:** J.P. will combine vocalization with pointing to request an object.
>
> **Short-Term Objective 2.2:** J.P. will increase phonological skills.

Short-Term Objective Justification Realization of the first short-term objective (e.g., combining J.P.'s vocalizations with his intentional gestures) should increase his communicative effectiveness. Paul (2001) indicated that effective intervention starts with what the child can do and takes it further. We know that J.P. can request objects through the use of pointing and eye gaze. We also know that J.P. can use some limited vocalizations ("buh," "bah," and "duh"). Children between 12 and 18 months typically combine gestures with vocalizations as they progress toward the combination of words and gestures. According to Owens (2001), children's first words fulfill previously expressed communicative intentions. Therefore it is reasonable to develop J.P.'s use of vocalization and word approximations to request objects. The vocalizations to be encouraged are those that include consonants. Whitehurst et al. (1992) indicated that vowel babble does not move the child toward speech, whereas consonant babble does. Therefore to build on what J.P. already does, his vocalizations with /b/ and/or /d/ will be promoted.

The second short-term objective focuses on increasing J.P.'s phonological skills. According to Layton (2000), problems with speech intelligibility are common among children with Down syndrome. J.P. has few vocalizations, a limited consonant inventory, and restricted syllable shape; therefore he is at risk for a continued expressive language delay and needs intervention targeted for this component of language. Paul (2001) indicated that "the primary goal of phonological intervention in the earliest stages of language development should be the enlargement of the consonant inventory and the range of syllable shapes the child can produce" (p. 276).

Strategy: Communication Form To facilitate J.P.'s use of requests, the language facilitator must keep a few things in mind, including the opportunities J.P. has to request and the type of response on the part of the language facilitator. In collaboration with the caregiver, specific daily events should be identified in which J.P. can be provided with multiple opportunities to request. The caregiver identified snack time as an event in which she would be willing to manipulate the environment, as well as to employ specific language facilitation techniques. Mrs. P. will set out cut pieces of banana and a drink. The caregiver will begin by modeling "want banana?" If J.P. points, the caregiver may want to wait for a vocalization instead of responding to J.P.'s communicative gesture. If J.P. does not respond initially, the caregiver can model "bahbah, banana," thus providing the more mature form.

Paul (2001) and Blacklin and Crais (1997) indicated that back-and-forth babbling games are effective for increasing the consonant inventory and syllable shape. It is suggested that the speech–language pathologist or caregiver imitate the child's babbling and continue doing so until the child imitates the adult's babbling. Once the back-and-forth game is established, the speech–language pathologist (or caregiver) introduces a new sound that is developmentally appropriate to the babble. In J.P.'s case, the next set of sounds to be introduced is velar consonants, /k/ and /g/. Bleile and Miller (1993) suggested that these velar consonants be facilitated either at the end of a syllable (VC) or after a front vowel (VC). Alternatively, sounds for which the child is stimulable may be incorporated. As noted in Chapter 3, Bleile (1995) suggested that when the focus of intervention with toddlers is on their phonological systems, the goals should be expansion of the phonetic inventory and syllable structure and targeting of stimulable sounds. J.P. imitated "lalala" when singing a song; thus the consonant "l" may be incorporated into the babbling games.

Communication Outcome 3

> Communication Outcome 3: J.P. will increase his semantic understanding and receptive communication skills.

Justification This communication outcome tries to ensure that J.P. has the necessary cognitive and linguistic skills before establishing an expressive communication outcome. Play, as noted in Chapter 3, is a link between the child's cognitive knowledge and the child's ability to use language. J.P. is currently using objects appropriately; however, it was noted during the assessment that J.P. was not interested in feeding or grooming a doll or stuffed animal. Therefore J.P.'s symbolic capabilities in play are not known. In addition, as noted in Chapter 3, as the child's language skill progresses to the use of first words (symbolic behavior), a parallel shift occurs in the child's play; he or she demonstrates symbolic play. The child pretends with realistic objects using conventional functions towards himself or herself. Therefore it is important to develop J.P.'s symbolic play skills while increasing his knowledge of words.

> Short-Term Objective 3.1: J.P. will understand a variety of nouns and actions.
>
> Short-Term Objective 3.2: J.P. will demonstrate single-sequence actions on objects.

Short-Term Objective Justification   The first short-term objective is designed to develop J.P.'s language comprehension as a basis for language expression. Olswang, Rodriguez, and Timler (1998) indicated that "receptive vocabulary in infants and toddlers who are developing typically is correlated with later word production" (p. 25). Thus the development of vocabulary comprehension is important in children with language delays. These authors further indicated that a receptive language delay of 6 months or longer has a poor prognosis and is indicative of the need for early intervention. Although J.P.'s language comprehension is not as delayed as other components of his language, development of comprehension is essential for the development of expressive language (Paul, 2001). It is critically important for the interventionist to develop J.P.'s understanding of early vocabulary items (nouns and verbs). To further develop J.P.'s receptive language abilities, the interventionist must develop his receptive vocabulary for objects and observed actions.

Layton (2000) reported that the play skills of children with Down syndrome follow a pattern of development similar to that of typically developing children. Symbolic play was also reported to develop in the same sequence for children with Down syndrome. Because there is a strong relationship between early symbolic play (action sequences on objects), it is crucial to develop J.P.'s symbolic play skills so that those skills might support and promote his use of spoken words. According to Yoder, Warren, and Hull (1995), intervention that included symbolic and combinatorial play correlated with increases in prelinguistic intentional requesting behavior.

Strategy: Language Comprehension and Symbolic Play   Layton (2000) reported that language intervention strategies employed with children with specific language deficits are effective for children with Down syndrome; therefore efforts to increase J.P.'s language comprehension should occur simultaneously with the development of his expressive language abilities. The language facilitator, caregiver, or speech–language pathologist should implement the techniques described in communication outcome 1 (e.g., following J.P.'s lead and using words in such a way as to provide names for objects and actions that are the focus of J.P.'s attention). The language facilitator should model language that gives J.P. information about objects, actions, and the relationships between objects and actions. Thus while engaged in everyday events (e.g., changing J.P.'s diaper, dressing him, or bathing him) the adult can use self-talk about what he or she is doing (e.g., take off shoes, take off socks, and take off pants), as well as parallel talk, to provide language for J.P.'s actions. The language should map the objects and actions as they occur in the natural setting (environment).

The language facilitator should engage in symbolic play with J.P. For example, repetition of everyday events can be replicated with a doll or stuffed animal. Thus J.P. and the language facilitator can give the doll a bath, dress the doll, and so forth. During this play activity the language facilitator can demonstrate the actions on the doll, as well as support J.P.'s ability to perform the actions on the doll. Once again, while engaged in these play activities the language facilitator should provide J.P. with appropriate language input.

INTERVENTION PLAN FOR BRANDON Z.

Communication Outcome 1

> Communication Outcome 1: B.Z. will improve his phonological skills.

Justification B.Z. exhibited an expressive and receptive language delay of 10 to 12 months and a significant delay in phonological development. According to Blacklin and Crais (1997), "from the early stages of word development, the child's phonology and lexicon are linked in a variety of ways" (p. 216). Therefore, this long-term communication outcome focuses on B.Z.'s speech production because it is imperative to increase the number and variety of phonemes Brandon produces to increase his lexicon. Whitehurst, Smith, Fischel, Arnold, and Lonigan (1991) indicated that it is important to strengthen the phonetic repertoire to increase the child's ability to acquire new words.

> Short-Term Objective 1.1: B.Z. will increase the number of front consonant sounds used.
>
> Short-Term Objective 1.2: B.Z. will increase his phonemic repertoire by expanding his syllable shapes.

Short-Term Objective Justification According to Blacklin and Crais (1997), there is general agreement in the literature about the "need for enhanced phoneme availability, syllable structure, mean length of utterance, lexical development, and syntagmatic distance (movement of the tongue from the front to the back of the mouth)" (p. 219). Thus the first short-term objective focuses on increasing the number and variety of consonant sounds used with a particular focus on front sounds. The second short-term objective is integrally related to the first; because of B.Z.'s limited consonant inventory, he will not be able to develop more complex syllable structures. As indicated earlier, phonological development has a strong influence on the early words young children produce (Blacklin & Crais, 1997). According to a variety of sources (Lindner, 1993; Stoel-Gammon, 1991), a typical 24-month-old can correctly produce the following consonant sounds: /t/, /p/, /b/, /m/, /n/, /k/, and /g/. The feature that is common to five of the seven sounds is that they are produced in the front of the mouth. B.Z. was producing a /d/ and limitedly a /b/ and /n/. It is essential for B.Z. to expand on his current abilities and produce additional front consonants. "Children often build their vocabulary with words having certain sounds, syllable structures and sound classes or sound features" (Blacklin and Crais, 1997, p. 217); therefore it is imperative to expand B.Z.'s consonant repertoire.

Stoel-Gammon (1991) noted that normally developing 2-year-olds are capable of producing a variety of syllable shapes. As reported in Chapter 3, Stoel-Gammon (1991) indicated that 97% of the 24-month-olds in her study used the syllable structure of CV. In addition, 97% of the children also used a syllable structure of CVC. Other syllable structures that were used included

CVCV ("baby," "doggie"; 79% of the children) and CVCVC ("pocket"; 65% of the children). B.Z.'s syllable shape was limited during the assessment; therefore, it is crucial that the interventionist expand this area to provide B.Z. with more flexibility in word production. Bolstering B.Z.'s use of his preferred CV syllable structure and introducing the use of VC syllables will add phonological complexity by encouraging front-to-back and back-to-front movements in order to facilitate CVC syllables (Blacklin & Crais, 1997).

Strategy: Phonological Skills A variety of techniques can be employed to facilitate sound production; however, the contexts and the activities in which the intervention occurs must incorporate the interests of the child, as well as the ongoing activities in the child's environments. The speech–language pathologist can work with the caregivers to adapt the environment in such a way that the primary interventionist can follow the child's lead in naturally occurring events. Modeling by the speech–language pathologist and caregiver can be implemented so that all items attended to by the child include the target phonemes and are in the appropriate syllable structure. For example, while playing with farm animals the speech–language pathologist or caregiver can model "moo" and other farm animal sounds. In addition, he or she can read a picture book about animals and say, for example, "the baby cow says moo." In addition, bubbles can be available for popping, providing multiple opportunities for the adult to model "pop."

Communication Outcome 2

> Communication Outcome 2: B.Z. will increase his expressive language skills.

Justification Children on average have a productive expressive lexicon of 55 words at 16 months, 225 words at 23 months, and 569 words at 30 months (Fenson, Dale, Resnick, Bates, Thal & Pethick, 1994). According to Paul (2001), children between the ages of 18 and 24 months use words and word combinations to express a variety of intents. B.Z. was able to produce 10 words, and when combining these words with his use of gestures he was able to express a variety of communicative intents. However, his use of words to express his communicative intents was significantly reduced.

> Short-Term Objective 2.1: B.Z. will use a single word to comment.
>
> Short-Term Objective 2.2: B.Z. will use a vocalization paired with a gesture to request an object.

Short-Term Objective Justification This first intervention outcome focuses on the priority of developing B.Z.'s expressive vocabulary, which is in accordance with Mrs. Z.'s desire to have Brandon talk like the other children. Brandon reportedly was using 7 to 10 word approximations, which provided evidence that he was capable of producing words. Using a few words is a good prognostic indicator that he could acquire additional words. In deciding on target words for Brandon, factors to consider include selecting words that are similar to those used by typically developing children (Paul, 2001), choosing words with potential for communicative effectiveness (Bloom & Lahey, 1978), and determining words based on their phonological composition and syllable shape (Paul, 2001). The interests of the child and the desired outcome of the caregiver should be taken into account. An overriding consideration is that the words targeted allow the child to meet his or her social and communicative goals.

With these considerations in mind, the interventionist selected the first short-term goal because it specifically focuses on a particular communicative function: commenting. Commenting was chosen as the first communicative function to help B.Z. develop single words because he was using word approximations to comment on objects (name people and objects).

The second short-term objective was chosen based on the typical progression of expressive language development in which the child pairs a gesture with a vocalization or a word approximation before relying on single words. B.Z. was using only eye gaze to request objects in his environment. B.Z.'s phonological repertoire and the first communicative outcome should be kept in mind when requesting is developed. This objective focuses on word approximations in combination with gestures because, according to Whitehurst, et al. (1991), phonological intervention is probably more motivating for the young child if it is in the context of teaching words.

Fey and Cleave (1990) indicated that the interventionist also should remember that providing intervention on a basic specific target, in this case request for objects, may result in enhanced performance in terms of goals that have not been directly targeted. Thus it is hoped that an increase in requests for action is seen.

Strategy: Form of Expressing Communicative Intent When facilitating expressive language, the speech–language pathologist should remember that a child is more likely to produce a word if that word consists of phonemes that are in the child's repertoire (Paul, 2001). Another consideration is the ease with which words can eventually be combined into short phrases.

B.Z. could produce /t/, /d/, and /n/ consistently; therefore, various home routines can be identified and the caregivers can be instructed to use the child-centered techniques of self-talk, modeling, expansion, and so forth to expose Brandon to words that were appropriate. For example, during a bath routine the targeted words—nose, toes, tummy, neck, ears, eyes—can be stressed by the caregiver and an interactive game of washing various body parts can be employed to provide B.Z. with a context in which to use the targeted vocabulary.

Joint book reading is a powerful tool to facilitate expressive language in young children (Crain-Thoreson & Dale, 1999; Kaiser, Hemmeter, Ostrosky, Fischer, Yoder & Keefer, 1996). Whitehurst, Arnold, Epstein, Angell, Smith & Fischel (1994) reported that joint book reading facilitates vocabulary growth. B.Z.'s caregivers and teachers will be given instruction in interactive book reading. Book reading is a natural time to comment on pictures, so this method in conjunction with the first strategy can be used to facilitate words for commenting. A book that presents a bath time or other nighttime routines can be used to expand and elaborate on that routine and use single words that are within B.Z.'s phonetic inventory.

To facilitate B.Z.'s use of single words and vocalizations to request, the communicative context may have to be manipulated for B.Z. to experience the state of needing an object. Wetherby and Prizant (1989) described a variety of "communicative temptations" that can be used to assess a child's ability to express various communicative intents. Lindner (1993) called these events "communicative enticers" or activities that encourage the child to request. Likewise the communicative temptations that are meant to elicit request behaviors can be modified and routinized to form the basis of an intervention context for eliciting request behavior. Thus a food container containing a favorite snack can be the catalyst for an event in which the caregiver gives B.Z. a piece of the snack, then closes the container tightly, hands it to B.Z., and waits. If B.Z. attempts to communicate, the caregiver should respond with the word that maps B.Z.'s request. The caregiver may have to encourage B.Z. to communicate; to accomplish this, a question such as "what do you want?" can be employed. If B.Z. hands the container back but does not verbalize, the caregiver can model "Oh, you want a cracker," with additional repetition of the word "cracker."

Communication Outcome 3

> Communication Outcome 3: B.Z. will increase his receptive language skills.

Justification The relationship between receptive and expressive language skills is not clear. However, Owens (2001) indicated that for the first 50 words comprehension precedes production. For B.Z. to become a functional communicator within the family structure (and in society as a whole), he must be able to comprehend language. Young children use their knowledge about familiar events to facilitate their responses. Familiar events provide scripts that aid comprehension. The goal in working on B.Z.'s comprehension abilities is to enable him to use both event knowledge and, eventually, linguistic knowledge to aid his comprehension. Therefore the initial step is to increase his world knowledge, as well as his word knowledge, so that he has multiple strategies to facilitate his response to language. The level of the child's involvement affects comprehension (Owens, 1999). Therefore B.Z. should be actively involved in the events so that he can make active associations between words and the nonlinguistic context (Paul, 1990). In addition, the repetitive nature of familiar routines will assist B.Z. by increasing his expectations and recall (Owens, 1999).

> Short-Term Objective 3.1: B.Z. will increase his knowledge of complex language by demonstrating knowledge of objects, locations, and actions.
>
> Short-Term Objective 3.2: B.Z. will increase his ability to understand simple directions (follow one- and two-step related commands that are contextually supported).

Short-Term Objective Justification To increase B.Z.'s understanding of complex language, knowledge of objects (such as ball, slide, swing), locations (on table, in box), and actions (such as eat, push, throw, hit, jump, kick, run) will be targeted. Intervention for B.Z.'s receptive language can be designed not only to facilitate his acquisition of specific target words but also to simultaneously facilitate his knowledge of the world. Exposing B.Z. to words to express the relationships between objects, events, and locations in the world will increase his knowledge of the specific target goals, as well as allow him to develop more sophisticated play and adaptive skills. Children learn by doing, so the child needs to actively engage in play that demonstrates the objects, actions, and relationships that have been targeted for intervention. After collaboration with B.Z.'s caregivers, specific child interests were identified that can serve as the basis of intervention, such as play activities in which B.Z. is given the opportunity to engage in natural learning. During a visit to the park, B.Z. is exposed to objects (balls, merry-go-round, swings), actions (because the toys all move), and locations ("up the slide," "climb the stairs," and so forth), all of which ensure exposure to complex language.

The second short-term objective is for B.Z. to understand simple directions. At first a child follows commands and directions with only one verb, and later those with two verbs. Therefore this short-term objective is tied to the first; for B.Z. to follow a command, comprehension of the objects and actions involved must be ensured. Lindner (1993) suggested that a child's ability to follow commands (directions) should be implemented within playful games.

Strategy: Receptive Language According to Cripe, Slentz, and Bricker (1993), children learn to associate objects, events, and people by repeatedly hearing the words while interacting with the environment. Weitzman (1992) indicated that the use of labels for objects, people, actions, and events helps the child build up a store of receptive language, which he or she will eventually use. Indirect language stimulation (ILS) is a child-centered technique whereby the caregiver or speech–language pathologist provides the appropriate linguistic markers for objects, events, and relationships in context as the child experiences them. Indirect language stimulation as described by Paul (2001) is a technique that is "especially appropriate for clients in the 18-36 month developmental level" (p. 275). Caregivers can be instructed on how to map linguistic form to referents that are found in play. The caregiver can use the techniques described in Chapter 7 to provide linguistic mappings for B.Z.'s involvement in play. Use of the child-centered input strategies will provide B.Z. with structured input. B.Z.'s participation in daily activities and activities of interest should be the focus of intervention for receptive language. B.Z.'s primary caregiver, his mother, reported that B.Z. particularly enjoys playing with trucks. Therefore, she was encouraged to do the following:

- Create a play routine in which a small figure is placed in the truck and drives it to the store, school, home, and so forth, to develop connections between B.Z.'s interests and word knowledge.
- Use language during this play routine that is repetitive and eventually develops into a script, so that B.Z. can use the nonlinguistic events to begin to decode the words used in the routine.
- Specifically, use expansion techniques.

Joint book reading is another way to develop receptive language skills. When looking at a book with B.Z., the language facilitator (caregiver or speech–language pathologist) can name the pictures in the book. An "all about me" book with real photos of favorite people, toys, and events can be an effective tool. A young child will enjoy looking at it repeatedly, and the language facilitator can provide an effective vehicle to map linguistic skills to world knowledge.

During playtime with familiar objects, the caregiver can be encouraged to ask B.Z. to demonstrate a familiar action. For example, during a wash-a-doll activity, B.Z. can be asked to wash the dolly's hair, wash the dolly's face, or open the shampoo. If B.Z. does not follow the direction, then the speech–language pathologist or caregiver should model the correct action.

REFERENCES

Blacklin, J., & Crais, E. R. (1997). A treatment protocol for young children at risk for severe expressive output disorders. *Seminars in Speech and Language 18*(3), 213-237.

Bleile, K. M. (1995). *Manual of articulation and phonological disorders.* San Diego: Singular.

Bleile, K., & Miller, S. (1993). Articulation and phonological disorders in toddlers with medical needs. In J. Bernthal (Ed.), *Articulatory and phonological disorders in special populations* (pp. 81-109). New York: Thieme.

Bloom, L., & Lahey, M. (1978). *Language development and language disorders.* New York: Wiley.

Crain-Thoreson, C., & Dale, P. S. (1999). Enhancing linguistic performance: Parents and teachers as book reading partners for children with language delays. *Topics in Early Childhood Special Education, 19,* 28-39.

Cripe, J., Slentz, K., & Bricker, D. (1993). *Assessment, evaluation, and programming system for infants and children, Vol. 2: AEPS curriculum for birth to three years.* Baltimore: Brookes.

Fenson, L., Dale, P. S., Reznick, J. S., Bates, E., Thal, D. J., & Pethick, S. J. (1994). Variability in early communicative development. *Monographs of the Society for Research in Child Development, 59*(5) Serial #242.

Fey, M. E., & Cleave, P. L. (1990). Early language intervention. *Seminars in Speech and Language, 11*(3), 165-181.

Kaiser, A. P., Hemmeter, M. L., Ostrosky, M. M., Fischer, R., Yoder, P., & Keefer, M. (1996). The effects of teaching parents to use responsive interaction strategies. *Topics in Early Childhood Special Education, 16*(3), 375-406.

Layton T. L. (2000). Young children with Down syndrome. In T. L. Layton, E. Crais, & L. R. Watson (Eds.), *Handbook of early language impairment in children: Nature* (pp. 193-231). Albany, NY: Delmar Thomson Learning.

Lindner, T. (1993). *Transdisciplinary play-based intervention: Guidelines for developing a meaningful curriculum for young children.* Baltimore: Brookes.

Olswang, L. B., Rodriguez, B., & Timler, G. (1998). Recommending intervention for toddlers with specific language learning difficulties: We may not have all the answers, but we know a lot. *American Journal of Speech–Language Pathology, 3*(7), 23-32.

Owens, R. E. (1999). *Language disorders: A functional approach to assessment and intervention* (3rd Ed.). Boston: Allyn & Bacon.

Owens, R. E. (2001). *Language development: An introduction* (5th Ed.). Boston: Allyn & Bacon.

Paul, R. (1990). Comprehension strategies: Interactions between world knowledge and the development of sentence comprehension. *Topics in Language Disorders, 10*(3), 63-75.

Paul, R. (2001). *Language disorders: From infancy through adolescence* (2nd Ed). St Louis, MO: Mosby.

Stoel-Gammon, C. (1991). Normal and disordered phonology in two-year olds. *Topics in Language Disorders, 11*(4), 21-32.

Weitzman, E. (1992). *Learning language and loving it.* Toronto: Hanen Center.

Wetherby, A., & Prizant, B. (1989). The expression of communicative intent: Assessment guidelines. *Seminars in Speech and Language, 10*(1), 77-91.

Whitehurst, G. J., Arnold, D. S., Epstein, J. N., Angell, A. L., Smith, M., & Fischel, J. E. (1994). A picture book reading intervention in day care and home for children from low-income families. *Developmental Psychology, 30*(5), 679-689.

Whitehurst, G. J., Fischel, J. E., Arnold, D. S., & Lonigan, C. L. (1992). Evaluating outcomes with children with expressive language delay. In S. Warren & J. Reichle (Eds.), *Causes and effects in communication and language intervention* (pp. 277-313). Baltimore: Brookes.

Whitehurst, G. J., Smith, M., Fischel, J. E., & Lonigan, C. L. (1991). The continuity of babble and speech in children with specific expressive language delay. *Journal of Speech and Hearing Research, 34*(5), 1121-1129.

Yoder, P. J., Warren, S. F., & Hull, L. (1995). Predicting children's response to prelinguistic communication intervention. *Journal of Early Intervention, 19*(1), 74-84.

Assessment Tools:
Birth to Age 3

COMMUNICATIVE AND SYMBOLIC BEHAVIOR SCALES

The Communicative and Symbolic Behavior Scales (CSBS) (Wetherby & Prizant, 1993) is a norm-referenced, standardized instrument that examines communicative, social-affective, and symbolic abilities of children 9 to 24 months old whose communicative abilities range from preverbal to verbal. Observation, interaction, and parent interview are included. The format of the *CSBS* is standard but flexible, and includes both unstructured and elicitation tasks. The scales also include a form for parents to complete after the assessment to validate the results gained by the professional. The scales include eight communicative temptations to determine communicative function and mode of expression, a series of play contexts to determine combinatorial and symbolic play abilities, and comprehension items.

COMMUNICATIVE AND SYMBOLIC BEHAVIOR SCALES DEVELOPMENTAL PROFILE

The *Communicative and Symbolic Behavior Scales Developmental Profile (CSBS DP)* (Wetherby & Prizant, 1998) is an easy-to-use, norm-referenced screening and evaluation tool designed to determine the communicative competence of children with functional language between 6 months and 24 months of age (normed on children aged 6 months to 6 years). The three components of this assessment tool are a communication checklist, a caregiver questionnaire, and a behavior sample taken while the child interacts with a parent present. The format of the *CSBS DP* involves the caregiver completing the communication checklist to determine if further evaluation is needed and, if so, answering a more in-depth caregiver questionnaire and behavior sample. The scale measures seven areas that are predictors of language impairment in young children: emotion and eye gaze, communication, gestures, sounds, words, understanding, and object use.

MACARTHUR COMMUNICATIVE DEVELOPMENT INVENTORIES

The *MacArthur Communicative Development Inventories (CDIs)* (Fenson et al., 1993) are norm-referenced parent report forms for assessing language and communication skills in infants and young children. The *CDI: Words and Gestures* (infant form) is designed for use with 8- to 16-month-old children.

The *CDI: Words and Sentences* (toddler form) is designed for use with 16- to 30-month-old children. Either form may be used with older, developmentally delayed children.

ROSSETTI INFANT TODDLER LANGUAGE SCALE

The *Rossetti Infant Toddler Language Scale* (Rossetti, 1990) was developed for children from birth to 3 years of age. It includes parent questionnaire and a criterion referenced test protocol to gather observed, elicited, and parent report information. Test protocol examines interaction-attachment (the cues and responses that reflect a reciprocal relationship between the caregiver and the child), pragmatics (the way the child uses language to communicate with and affect others), gesture (the child's use of gestures to express thoughts and intent prior to the consistent use of spoken language), play (the changes in a child's play that reflect the development of representational thought), language comprehension (the child's understanding of verbal language with and without linguistic cues), and language expression (the child's use of preverbal and verbal behaviors to communicate with others). The parent questionnaire includes questions about concern, interaction, and communication development, and a vocabulary checklist (for produced and understood words).

RECEPTIVE-EXPRESSIVE EMERGENT LANGUAGE SCALE III

The *Receptive-Expressive Emergent Language Scale III (REEL-III)* (Bzoch, League, & Brown, 2003) is a standardized test that uses an interview format and investigates both receptive and expressive language behaviors. This instrument covers the age range from birth to 36 months. The child's performance is scored as typically exhibited, emerging, or not exhibited. The examiner scores high-frequency behaviors and arranges them into an ordinal sequence. Scores for receptive language age, expressive language age, and combined language age are produced. The third edition includes a new subtest, Inventory of Vocabulary Words. The third edition also has revised norms based on the 2000 U.S. census.

SEQUENCED INVENTORY OF COMMUNICATIVE DEVELOPMENT–REVISED

The *Sequenced Inventory of Communicative Development–Revised (SICD-R)* (Hedrick, Prather, & Tobin, 1984) assesses communication skills of infants, toddlers, and preschoolers from 4 months to 4 years of age. The areas assessed are awareness of environmental sounds and speech sounds, discrimination of environmental sounds and speech sounds, understanding, initiation of communication, imitation of communication, and response to communication. Items are assigned age levels based on the performance of normally developing children included in the standardization sample. Scores in receptive and expressive communication ages are produced and can be compared to the chronological or mental age, or both, of the child.

PRESCHOOL LANGUAGE SCALE–4

The *Preschool Language Scale–4 (PLS-4)* (Zimmerman, Steiner, & Pond, 2002) is a highly structured but flexible scale based on normative findings represent-ing the 2000 U.S. Census. The scale's norms are based on children from birth to 6 years 11 months of age. The norms are presented at 3-month intervals from 0 to 11 months, at 6-month intervals from 1 year to 4 years, and at 12-month intervals for 5 and 6 years of age. The scale assesses attention, vocal development, social communication, semantics (including vocabulary and concepts), structure (including syntax and morphology), and integrative thinking skills. The test also includes optional measures, which include an articulation screener, a language sample form and checklist, and a caregiver questionnaire. The caregiver questionnaire is designed to enable caregivers to share their knowledge of the child's typical communication at home. The child can receive credit for an item if the behavior was spontaneous, elicited, or by caregiver response. A Spanish edition of this assessment tool is also available.

ASSESSING LINGUISTIC BEHAVIORS

The *Assessing Linguistic Behaviors (ALB)* (Olswang, Stoel-Gammon, Coggins, & Carpenter, 1987) protocol was designed for use with children functioning below the age of 2 years who are at risk for or suspected of impaired language development. It includes five scales. The first scale, the Cognitive Antecedents to Word Meaning Scale, was designed to examine the cognitive skills for three early emerging semantic notions and their related pragmatic functions (Nomination, Agent, Location). The second scale, the Play Scale, examines the child's practice play during the first year of the sensorimotor period. The child's actions toward objects and the child's symbolic play are observed. The Communicative Intent Scale is the third scale. This scale is a criterion-referenced measure of a child's intentional communication. The fourth scale is the Language Comprehension Scale. The final scale is the Language Production Scale, which was designed to examine the vocalizations of children aged 9 to 24 months. The scale is divided into two major parts: one focusing on prelinguistic utterances (babbling) and the other on meaningful speech (linguistic productions).

REFERENCES

Bzoch, K. R., League, R., & Brown, V. (2003). *Receptive-Expressive Emergent Language Scale* (3rd Ed.). Dallas, TX: ProEd.

Fenson, L., Dale, P. S., Reznick, J. S., Thal, D., Bates, E., Hartung, J. P., Pethick, S. & Reilly, J. (1993). *MacArthur Communicative Development Inventories: User's guide and technical manual*. San Diego: Singular.

Hedrick, D. L, Prather, E. M., & Tobin, A. R. (1984). *Sequenced inventory of communication development* (Revised ed.). Seattle: University of Washington Press.

Olswang, L. B., Stoel-Gammon, C., Coggins, T. E., & Carpenter, R. L. (1987). *Assessing linguistic behaviors.* Seattle: University of Washington Press.

Rossetti, L. (1990). *Infant toddler Language Scale.* East Moline, IL: Lingua Systems Inc.

Wetherby, A. M., & Prizant, B. M. (1993). *Communicative and Symbolic Behavior Scales.* Itasca, IL: Riverside.

Wetherby, A. M., & Prizant, B. M. (1998). *Communication and Symbolic Behavior Scales Developmental Profile.* Baltimore: Brooks Publishing Company.

Zimmerman, I., Steiner, V., & Pond, R. (2002). *Preschool Language Scale–4 (PLS-4).* Austin, TX: Psychological Corporation.

I N D E X

Page numbers followed by b indicate boxes ; f, figures; t, tables.